1000 EMQs for PLAB
based on current exams

Second Edition

Sherif W Helmy MBBCh (Hons), MRCP (UK)

GP Registrar
Kent, Surrey and Sussex Deanery

Radcliffe Publishing
Oxford • San Francisco

Radcliffe Publishing Ltd
18 Marcham Road
Abingdon
Oxon OX14 1AA
United Kingdom

www.radcliffe-oxford.com
Electronic catalogue and worldwide online ordering facility.

_____

British Library Cataloguing in Publication Data

A catalogue record for this book is available from the British Library.

ISBN 1 85775 676 2

Typeset by Richard Powell Editorial and Production Services, Basingstoke, Hants
Printed and bound by TJ International Ltd, Padstow, Cornwall

Contents

Foreword   Iain Murray-Lyon   *vii*
About the author   *viii*
Introduction   *ix*

Themes   **1**

Breathlessness   3
Liver disease   4
Causes of haematemesis   5
Neurological disorders   6
Mass in the right iliac fossa   7
Investigating the biliary system   8
Causes of pneumonia   9
Anaemia   10
Operations in gynaecology and their indications   11
Ovarian tumours   12
Causes of acute pancreatitis   13
Cardiac lesions   14
Skin rash   15
Rectal bleeding in children   16
Arthritis   17
Genetics   18
Breast cancer   19
Lump in the groin   20
Causes of clubbing   21
Skin lesions   22
Operations in gynaecology and their indications   23
Urinary problems in women   24
Chest radiography findings in congenital heart diseases   25
Paediatric neurological disorders   26
Causes of syncope   27
Autoantibodies   28
Visual field defects   29
Renal calculi   30
Malnutrition and malabsorption   31
Adverse effects of medications   32
Pelvic pain   33
Staging of malignant tumours   34
Pulmonary diseases in children   35
Investigating pulmonary diseases in children   36
Adverse effects of medications   37
Liver diseases   38
Management of endometriosis   39

Investigating amenorrhoea	40
Laryngeal carcinoma	41
Thyrotoxicosis	42
Chest radiography findings	43
Anaemia	44
Haematological diseases in children	45
Paediatric oncology	46
ECG findings	47
Psychiatric disorders	48
Endocrine tumours	49
Jaundice	50
Causes of confusion	51
Drug overdose	52
Causes of haemoptysis	53
Human leucocytic antigens	54
Therapeutics	55
Amenorrhoea	56
Chest pain	57
Cerebrovascular disease	58
Lower limb ischaemia	59
Thyroid cancer	60
Inborn errors of metabolism	61
Neurological disorders	62
Renal impairment	63
Radiological investigations	64
Vaginal bleeding	65
Management of bleeding	66
Vascular disease	67
Skeletal pain	68
Breathlessness	69
Renal impairment	70
Investigating infertility	71
Teratogenic infections during pregnancy	72
Thyroid disorders	73
Infections	74
Investigating gastrointestinal disorders	75
Management of myasthenia gravis	76
Rheumatology	77
Sexually transmitted diseases	78
Adverse effects of medications	79
Anaesthesia during labour	80
Malabsorption	81
Congenital cardiac lesions	82
Management of gastrointestinal disorders	83
Blood supply to the brain	84
Chest pain in pregnancy	85
Blood film	86
Arthritis	87
Electrolyte imbalance	88

Dermatomes	89
Cranial nerves	90
Clinical features of AIDS	91
Physical signs of cardiac lesions	92
Haematological diseases	93
Diarrhoea	94
Thyroid function tests	95
Rheumatology	96
Physical signs of congenital heart diseases	97
Management of thoracic disorders	98
Renal pathology	99
Tumour markers	100
Tumour markers	101
Neurological disorders	102
Vasculitis	103
Acute abdominal pain	105
Risk factors for malignancies	107
Haematuria	108
Genetic disorders	109
Metabolic disturbances	110
Erythropoietin level	111
Immunodeficiency disorders	112
Investigations during pregnancy	113
Bone profile interpretation	114
Amenorrhoea	115
Abdominal pain	116
Rectal bleeding	117
Eye drops	118
Urinary symptoms in children	119
Viral infections in children	120
Haematemesis	121
Methods of contraception	122
Pupillary abnormalities	123
Monitoring of medication	124
Hoarseness of voice	125
Milestones in children	126
Prescribing medication in pregnancy	127
Visual problems	128
Muscle weakness	129
Physical signs in ophthalmology	130
Dysphagia	131
Psychiatric illness	132
ECG findings in arrhythmias and conduction defects	133
Interpretation of blood results	134
Arthritis	135
Vitamin deficiency	136
Bleeding in pregnancy	137
Mode of inheritance	138
Management of labour	139

Classification of medication in psychotherapy   140
Neonatal jaundice   141
Physical signs in dermatology   142
Neck swellings   143
Prescribing antimicrobials   144
Chromosomal abnormalities   145
Menorrhagia   146
Choice of contraception   147
Haematuria   148
Bacterial infections   149
Earache   150
Differential diagnosis of ectopic pregnancy   151
Infectious diseases   152
Driving regulations for group 1 drivers   153
Scrotal swelling   154
Prescribing medication in renal failure   155
Investigating vaginal bleeding   156
Prescribing medication in chronic liver disease   157
Electrolyte imbalance   158
Choice of analgesia   160
Management of angina   161
Causes of mouth ulcers   162
Abdominal discomfort   163
Medical syndromes   164
Seizures   165
Red eyes   166
Thoracic tumours   167
Headache   168
Vaginal bleeding   169
Investigating a neck swelling   170
Abdominal pain   171
Prescribing antimicrobials   172
Liver diseases   173
Carcinogens   174

Answers   **177**

Appendix: Normal values   *184*

Foreword

Dr Sherif Helmy is a physician with wide experience, and he has applied his knowledge and skills to great effect in preparing this excellent book which will, I am sure, prove to be of immense value to those preparing for the PLAB exam. It is topic-based, covering a wide range of subjects. The questions are all clinically relevant to day-to-day practice, and clearly formulated. Working carefully through this book should form an important part of the process of preparation for the exam and I am very happy to recommend it.

Dr Iain Murray-Lyon, MD, FRCP, FRCP(Ed)
Honorary Consultant Physician and Gastroenterologist to
Chelsea and Westminster Hospital
London SW10 9NH

About the author

Sherif Helmy is currently a GP Registrar in Surrey. He trained in several teaching hospitals in London, Surrey and the Midlands. He has a special interest in Diabetes and Endocrinology.

Introduction to the revised edition

This book aims to provide a useful tool for preparing for the PLAB test. It contains 1000 EMQs (extended matching questions) written in the same format as the actual test.

EMQs in this book are carefully selected to cover all clinical specialities. Most of the EMQs are similar to those in the actual test. You will notice that certain topics are covered more extensively than others, in view of their clinical relevance.

It is of vital importance to concentrate on all the details given in questions, e.g. age, past medical history and results of investigations. Such details can significantly influence the answers.

The best way in which to maximise the benefit obtained from this book is to read more about the topics covered from a reference book, as this book is not intended for use as reference.

Finally, I wish all candidates sitting the PLAB test the best of luck on the day and a bright medical career in the UK.

Sherif Helmy
London, January 2004

Themes

Theme: Breathlessness

Options

A. Inhaled foreign body
B. Anaemia
C. Pulmonary oedema
D. Bronchogenic carcinoma
E. Extrinsic allergic alveolitis
F. Pneumothorax

G. Pulmonary embolism
H. Pneumonia
I. Bronchial asthma
J. Pleural effusion
K. Cryptogenic fibrosing alveolitis

Instructions

For each case, choose the single most appropriate diagnosis from the above list of options. Each option may be used once, more than once or not at all.

1. A 52-year-old woman on HRT presents with swollen left calf, chest pain and shortness of breath.
2. A 78-year-old man has been short of breath for a few weeks. His chest radiography shows a right basal shadow rising towards the axilla.
3. A 45-year-old woman presents with progressive breathlessness and cyanosis. Clinical examination reveals clubbing and bilateral inspiratory crackles.
4. A 27-year-old farmer presented with fever, malaise, cough and breathlessness, which he had had for a few days. His symptoms were worse in the evening. Clinical examination demonstrated coarse end-inspiratory crackles.
5. A 34-year-old tall slim porter presents with sudden-onset chest pain and breathlessness. He has had similar episodes in the past.
6. A 76-year-old man presents with acute breathlessness, cough, frothy blood-stained sputum and palpitations. He is apyrexial. ECG shows sinus tachycardia.

Theme: Liver disease

Options

A. Wilson's disease
B. Sclerosing cholangitis
C. Primary biliary cirrhosis
D. Haemochromatosis
E. Galactosaemia
F. Gaucher's disease

G. Dubin–Johnson syndrome
H. Gilbert's syndrome
I. Hepatocellular carcinoma
J. Pancreatic carcinoma
K. Chronic active hepatitis

Instructions

For each case, choose the single most appropriate diagnosis from the above list of options. Each option may be used once, more than once or not at all.

7. A 48-year-old man presents with a dull aching pain in the right hypochondrium, which has had for 3 weeks. Other complaints include impotence, arthritis, lethargy and weight loss.

8. A 47-year-old alcoholic presents with weight loss, fever, ascites and pain in the right hypochondrium. Abdominal ultrasound shows a focal lesion in a cirrhotic liver. Serum AFP is grossly elevated.

9. A 41-year-old man with known ulcerative colitis presented with progressive abdominal pain and itching. On examination he was jaundiced.

10. A 35-year-old woman presented with jaundice and painless de-pigmented patches on her hands, neck and face. On examination multiple spider naevi were noted.

11. A 4-week-old baby was seen with vomiting, diarrhoea and failure to thrive. On examination there was hepatomegaly.

12. A 27-year-old nurse presented with jaundice and pruritus a few weeks after starting oral contraceptive pills. She gave no history of exposure to halothane, and hepatitis serology was negative. Liver functions tests were normal but urine showed bilirubinuria.

Theme: Causes of haematemesis

Options

A. Duodenal ulcer
B. Vascular malformation
C. Mallory–Weiss tear
D. Oesophageal varices
E. Gastric carcinoma
F. Crohn's disease

G. Oesophageal carcinoma
H. Haemophilia
I. Gastric ulcer
J. Oesophagitis
K. Meckel's diverticulum

Instructions

For each case, choose the single most appropriate diagnosis from the above list of options. Each option may be used once, more than once or not at all.

13. A 53-year-old unemployed alcoholic presents with haematemesis, a history of alcoholic liver disease and ascites.
14. A 77-year-old man with a history of dysphagia mainly to solid food and weight loss for 4 months.
15. A 59-year-old bank manager, with a long history of indigestion, presents with haematemesis, severe constant epigastric pain and weight loss.
16. A 34-year-old man presents with haematemesis, a history of back pain, arthritis, diarrhoea and weight loss.
17. A 37-year-old labourer presented to A&E with haematemesis after an episode of severe coughing. On examination he was very drunk and drowsy but there were no signs of chronic liver disease.
18. A 42-year-old secretary presents with haematemesis. She also complains of epigastric pain, which usually occurs at night. The pain is relieved by antacids and is worse when she is hungry.

Theme: Neurological disorders

Options

A. Subdural haematoma
B. Guillain–Barré syndrome
C. Frontal lobe abscess
D. Brain stem haemorrhage
E. Petit mal epilepsy
F. Multiple sclerosis
G. Benign intracranial hypertension

H. Arnold–Chiari malformation
I. Meningitis
J. Normal pressure hydrocephalus
K. Motor neuron disease

Instructions

For each case, choose the single most appropriate diagnosis from the above list of options. Each option may be used once, more than once or not at all.

19. A 37-year-old engineer was started on diuretics three months ago for hypertension (180/110). A few weeks later he was admitted to A&E with vomiting, acute vertigo and gross incoordination. On examination there was bilateral nystagmus.

20. A 78-year-old hypertensive woman is referred for fluctuating level of consciousness. On examination her blood pressure is 175/110, fundus examination shows some hypertensive changes, her reflexes are bilaterally brisk and her plantars are upgoing.

21. A 26-year-old presents with a week's history of headache and diplopia. On examination she is obese and fundoscopy shows bilateral papilloedema.

22. A 28-year-old diplomat presented with sudden blurring of the left eye. A week earlier he noted progressive clumsiness of the right hand. A few months earlier he had had an episode of left leg stiffness that resolved spontaneously.

23. A 19-year-old soldier is brought semiconscious into A&E. He has been complaining of severe headache and vomiting of one day duration. On examination there is widespread maculopapular rash all over his body.

24. A 36-year-old previously fit man developed a flu-like illness which was followed 2 days later by burning pain in both legs. He later developed urinary retention and diplopia. On examination his straight leg raising test was positive bilaterally, ocular mobility was limited bilaterally but sensation was intact.

Theme: Mass in the right iliac fossa

Options

A. Appendicular mass
B. Tuberculosis
C. Crohn's disease
D. Ulcerative colitis
E. Caecal carcinoma
F. Lymphoma

G. Ectopic kidney
H. Tubo-ovarian mass
I. Ectopic pregnancy
J. Intussusception
K. Volvulus

Instructions

For each case, choose the single most appropriate diagnosis from the above list of options. Each option may be used once, more than once or not at all.

25. A 20-year-old Somali man presents with a 2-month history of weight loss, fever and mass in the right iliac fossa (Hb 10 g/dl, WCC 13 000/mm$_3$, ESR 90 mm/h).
26. A 20-year-old Greek man presents with a 4-month history of weight loss, fever, night sweats and right-sided abdominal pain. The pain usually follows alcohol intake. Clinical examination reveals a mass in the right iliac fossa.
27. A 70-year-old woman presents with nausea, increasing dyspepsia and a mass in the right iliac fossa (Hb 9.8 g/dl, MCV 65 fl).
28. A 25-year-old man is found to have a mobile mass in the right iliac fossa during a routine medical examination for insurance purposes.
29. A 25-year-old man presents with a 3-month history of central colicky abdominal pain associated with occasional vomiting and diarrhoea. A barium follow-through demonstrates the string sign of the terminal ileum, and clinical examination reveals a mass in the right iliac fossa.

Theme: Investigating the biliary system

Options

A. Endoscopic retrograde cholangiopancreatography (ERCP) and sphincterotomy
B. Percutaneous transhepatic cholangiography (PTC)
C. HIDA scan
D. Computed tomography (CT) scan
E. Oral cholecystogram
F. Serum CA 19-9
G. Barium follow-through
H. Plain abdominal radiography
I. Magnetic resonance imaging (MRI)
J. Oesophagogastro-duodenoscopy
K. Laparoscopy

Instructions

For each case, choose the single most appropriate method of investigation from the above list of options. Each option may be used once, more than once or not at all.

30. A 59-year-old man presents with obstructive jaundice. Ultrasound scan shows no gallstones. The liver appears normal and the common bile duct measures 12 mm in diameter. His past medical history includes partial gastrectomy 15 years ago for peptic ulcer.

31. A 45-year-old woman presents with upper abdominal pain and obstructive jaundice. The gallbladder is not palpable clinically. Ultrasound shows gallstones and a dilated common bile duct (diameter = 15 mm).

32. A 50-year-old obese woman presents with acute upper abdominal pain. Examination demonstrates pyrexia, tachycardia and tenderness in the right upper abdomen. An erect chest radiograph reveals no free intraperitoneal gas. Ultrasound fails to confirm the clinical diagnosis of acute cholecystitis.

33. A 70-year-old woman presents with obstructive jaundice and a palpable gallbladder. Ultrasound shows a dilated common bile duct and enlargement of the pancreatic head. Her past medical history includes Polya gastrectomy for a bleeding peptic ulcer.

Theme: Causes of pneumonia

Options

A. Staphylococcus aureus
B. Cryptococcus
C. Streptococcus pneumoniae
D. Legionella pneumophila
E. Mycobacterium avium-
   intracellulare

F. Mycoplasma pneumoniae
G. Pneumocystis carinii
H. Chlamydia psittaci
I. Escherichia coli
J. Pseudomonas aeruginosa
K. Mycobacterium tuberculosis

Instructions

For each case, choose the single most appropriate causative organism from the above list of options. Each option may be used once, more than once or not at all.

34. A 37-year-old man presents with dyspnoea, cough, weight loss and night sweats. His chest radiograph shows diffuse bilateral infiltration.
35. A 48-year-old man presents with fever, rigors, headache and diarrhoea. He has recently been on holiday abroad. His chest x-ray shows consolidation.
36. A 24-year-old man presents with dry cough, skin manifestations, and bone and muscle aches. His chest radiograph shows widespread patchy shadows. Blood tests show evidence of haemolysis.
37. A 45-year-old farmer presents with flu-like illness, anorexia and dry cough. His chest radiograph shows patchy consolidation.
38. A 41-year-old drug abuser presents with fever, cough and breathlessness. This was preceded by viral influenza. Chest radiograph shows multiple abscesses.
39. A 14-year-old student with cystic fibrosis rapidly deteriorated and developed acute respiratory failure while in hospital.

Theme: Anaemia

Options

A. Iron deficiency anaemia
B. Spherocytosis
C. Autoimmune haemolytic anaemia
D. Aplastic anaemia
E. Sideroblastic anaemia
F. Pernicious anaemia

G. Anaemia of chronic disease
H. Thalassaemia major
I. Glucose-6-phosphate dehydrogenase deficiency
J. Folate deficiency anaemia
K. Sickle cell anaemia

Instructions

For each patient with anaemia described below, choose the single most appropriate diagnosis from the above list of options. Each option may be used once, more than once or not at all.

40. A 49-year-old radiographer presented with pallor, recurrent infections and epistaxis.
41. A 46-year-old epileptic on phenytoin presents with marked pallor.
42. A 14-year-old girl presented with fatigue. Her father was diagnosed in his youth as having recurrent anaemia. On examination, she is pale with a tinge of jaundice. The tip of her spleen is palpable.
43. A 78-year-old man presents with night fever, night sweats, easy fatiguability and pallor. On examination he has generalised lymphadenopathy and a large spleen.
44. A 12-year-old Greek boy with dysmorphic features was treated for 8 weeks with oral iron for anaemia without response. His blood film was dimorphic.
45. A 29-year-old man who is being treated for ulcerative colitis presents with pallor. His blood film shows reticulocytosis, fragmentation and Heinz bodies.

Theme: Operations in gynaecology and their indications

Options

A. Oophorectomy

B. Wertheim's hysterectomy

C. Dilatation and curettage

D. Ovarian cystectomy

E. Colporrhaphy

F. Myomectomy

G. Abdominal tubal ligation

H. Ventrosuspension

I. Manchester repair

J. Salpingectomy

K. Sling operation

Instructions

For each indication, choose the single most appropriate operation from the above list of options. Each option may be used once, more than once or not at all.

46. Stage I and II carcinoma of the cervix.

47. Symptomatic fibroids when the uterus is to be preserved for pregnancy.

48. Ectopic tubal pregnancy.

49. Sterilisation.

50. Benign ovarian cysts.

51. Symptomatic retroverted uterus.

Theme: Ovarian tumours

Options

A. Mucinous cystadenoma
B. Corpus luteum cysts
C. Endometrial cysts
D. Teratoma
E. Primary ovarian carcinoma
F. Serous cystadenoma
G. Retention cysts
H. Arrhenoblastoma
I. Ovarian fibroma
J. Theca cell tumour
K. Polycystic ovaries

Instructions

For each description, select the single most appropriate diagnosis from the above list of options. Each option may be used once, more than once or not at all.

52. The most common virilising tumour of the ovary. Secretes androgens.
53. Large multi-cavity ovarian cyst, filled with thick fluid. It may reach a huge size occupying the whole peritoneal cavity.
54. Single-cavity ovarian cyst, filled with watery fluid. Often bilateral. Potentially malignant.
55. Small, solid and hard, white benign tumour. Usually unilateral. May be associated with ascites and pleural effusion.
56. May contain sebaceous fluid, hair and teeth. May be benign or malignant.
57. Causes excessive oestrogen production. May occur at any age causing precocious puberty in children, metrorrhagia in adults and postmenopausal bleeding in older women.

Theme: Causes of acute pancreatitis

Options

A. Gallstones
B. Hypertriglyceridaemia
C. Mumps
D. Alcohol
E. Polyarteritis nodosa
F. Hypothermia

G. Cystic fibrosis
H. Pancreatic carcinoma
I. Iatrogenic
J. Thiazide diuretics
K. Hypercalcaemia

Instructions

For each case of acute pancreatitis described below, choose the single most appropriate diagnosis from the above list of options. Each option may be used once, more than once or not at all.

58. A 10-year-old girl with a history of recurrent chest infections and sinusitis presents with acute abdominal pain.
59. A 45-year-old obese woman with a history of recurrent pain in the right hypochondrium.
60. A 38-year-old driver presenting with recurrent central abdominal pain, diarrhoea and bleeding per rectum. Three weeks earlier, he had had a flu-like illness with productive cough and myalgia. Chest examination shows bilateral inspiratory wheezes.
61. A 65-year-old man presenting with progressive jaundice, anorexia and weight loss.
62. A 49-year-old woman presenting with polyuria, haematuria, abdominal pain and bone aches. On examination, her blood pressure is 170/100.
63. A 12-year-old student presenting with fever, anorexia, headache, malaise and trismus.

Theme: Cardiac lesions

Options

A. Mitral stenosis
B. Atrial septal defect
C. Fallot's tetralogy
D. Aortic stenosis
E. Hypertrophic
   cardiomyopathy

F. Mitral regurgitation
G. Tricuspid stenosis
H. Aortic regurgitation
I. Tricuspid regurgitation
J. Pulmonary stenosis
K. Ventricular septal defect

Instructions

For each set of clinical findings, choose the single most appropriate diagnosis from the above list of options. Each option may be used once, more than once or not at all.

64. Slow rising carotid pulse, prominent left ventricular impulse, ejection click, ejection systolic murmur and fourth heart sound.
65. Bounding carotid pulse, laterally displaced apex, ejection systolic murmur, early diastolic murmur and third heart sound.
66. Jerky carotid pulse, dominant 'a' wave in jugular venous pulse, double apical impulse, ejection systolic murmur at the base and pansystolic murmur at the apex.
67. Elevated jugular venous pressure, early diastolic opening snap, mid-diastolic murmur and loud first heart sound.
68. Elevated jugular venous pressure, displaced apex, pansystolic murmur at the apex and third heart sound.
69. Loud pansystolic murmur at the left lower sternal area, mid-diastolic flow murmur at the apex and loud second heart sound.

Theme: Skin rash

Options

A. Scabies
B. Measles
C. Cellulitis
D. Rubella
E. Roseola infantum
F. Erythema infectiosum

G. Varicella
H. Kawasaki disease
I. Rocky Mountain spotted fever
J. Scarlet fever
K. Meningococcal meningitis

Instructions

For each case, choose the single most appropriate diagnosis from the above list of options. Each option may be used once, more than once or not at all.

70. A 4-year-old boy presents with a vesicular rash that appears in crops.
71. A 5-year-old girl presented with a rash that started as a marked erythema of the cheeks.
72. A 14-year-old girl presents with intensely pruritic rash with pustules. On examination, the rash is generalised but is more in the folds between the fingers and toes.
73. A 6-year-old boy was admitted with fever and maculopapular rash. His mother reported that the rash first started on the face then became generalised. On examination, there is palpable cervical and occipital lymphadenopathy.
74. A 9-year-old boy presents with conjunctivitis and maculopapular rash. The rash started on the head and spread downwards.
75. An 18-month-old girl is admitted to A&E with a 6 hour history of fever and lethargy. On examination, her temperature is 38.9°C, blood pressure is 70/40, respiratory rate is 30 and pulse is 120. Examination also reveals a full fontanelle and a petechial rash.

Theme: Rectal bleeding in children

Options

A. Meckel's diverticulum
B. Eosinophilic colitis
C. Intussusception
D. Haemolytic–uraemic syndrome
E. Lymphonodular hyperplasia
F. Juvenile polyps
G. Ulcerative colitis
H. Crohn's disease
I. Haemorrhoids
J. Hirschsprung's disease
K. Anal fissure

Instructions

For each case, choose the single most appropriate diagnosis from the above list of options. Each option may be used once, more than once or not at all.

76. A 15-month-old boy is admitted to A&E shocked. There is no history of diarrhoea, but he has been passing large amounts of melanotic stool. On examination, he is anaemic.
77. A 4-year-old girl presents with bloody diarrhoea and crampy abdominal pain. Blood tests show anaemia and thrombocytopenia.
78. A 5-week-old infant presents with scanty streaks of fresh blood mixed with normal-coloured stools.
79. A 7-year-old boy presents with streaks of fresh blood on the side of normal-coloured stools and drops of fresh blood in the toilet. There is no history of abdominal or rectal pain.
80. A 3-year-old boy is admitted to A&E after passing several grossly bloody stools. There is no history of abdominal pain, fever or vomiting. On examination, he is markedly pale.
81. A 12-year-old girl presented with a 4-week history of rectal bleeding and frequent loose motions. She reported lower abdominal cramping during defaecation but denied fever, rash, weight loss, arthritis or vomiting. Investigations showed anaemia but normal ESR, albumin and liver enzymes.

Theme: Arthritis

Options

A. Rheumatoid arthritis
B. Psoriatic arthropathy
C. Systemic lupus erythematosus
D. Septic arthritis
E. Sero-negative arthritis

F. Pyrophosphate arthropathy
G. Haemarthrosis
H. Osteoarthritis
I. Gout
J. Hyperparathyroidism
K. Erythema nodosum

Instructions

For each case, choose the single most appropriate diagnosis from the above list of options. Each option may be used once, more than once or not at all.

82. A 77-year-old woman presents with pain and varus deformity of both knees. She also complains of pain in both hips and hands.
83. A 72-year-old woman presents with pain in both knees. Knee radiography show a rim of calcification of the lateral meniscus.
84. A 30-year-old woman presents with pain and morning stiffness of the small joints of both hands.
85. A 30-year-old flight attendant presents with gritty eyes and painful knees especially during standing. He has just returned from Thailand.
86. A 78-year-old man presented with pain and swelling of the left first metatarsal joint. He was started on thiazide diuretics 3 weeks earlier.
87. A 22-year-old soldier previously fit, presents with a red hot tender swollen knee. Leg muscles show marked spasm.

Theme: Genetics

Options

A. Schizophrenia
B. Coeliac disease
C. Vitamin D resistant rickets
D. Cystic fibrosis
E. Peptic ulcer
F. Familial adenomatous polyposis

G. Turner's syndrome
H. Frontal baldness
I. Rheumatoid arthritis
J. Duchenne muscular dystrophy
K. Hodgkin's lymphoma

Instructions

For each mode of inheritance, choose the single most appropriate disorder from the above list of options. Each option may be used once, more than once or not at all.

88. Autosomal dominant.
89. Autosomal recessive.
90. X-linked dominant.
91. X-linked recessive.
92. Sex-linked inheritance.
93. Polygenic inheritance.

Theme: Breast cancer

Options

A. Chemotherapy, LHRH analogues and bisphosphonates
B. Simple mastectomy
C. Tamoxifen
D. Radiotherapy
E. Patey's mastectomy
F. Wide local excision combined with axillary dissection plus radiotherapy and tamoxifen
G. Radical mastectomy
H. Expectant management
I. Excision biopsy and cytology

Instructions

For each case, choose the single most appropriate management from the above list of options. Each option may be used once, more than once or not at all.

94. A 70-year-old woman presents with a 2 cm lump in the upper outer quadrant of the right breast. The lump does not involve the skin and is mobile. Fine needle aspiration cytology reveals malignant cells. Mammography shows a speculate lesion corresponding to the lump.
95. A 40-year-old woman is found to have a widespread micro-calcification during screening mammography. A stereotactic cone biopsy reveals a low grade ductal carcinoma in situ.
96. A 35-year-old woman presents with a 4 cm carcinoma of the left breast and multiple bone metastases in the pelvis.
97. A 95-year-old woman presents with a locally advanced carcinoma of the left breast. The tumour is ER positive.

Theme: Lump in the groin

Options

A. Inguinal hernia
B. Femoral hernia
C. Saphenovarix
D. Spigelian hernia
E. Hydrocele

F. Inguinal lymphadenopathy
G. Haematocele
H. Femoral artery aneurysm
I. Pantaloon hernia

Instructions

For each case, choose the single most appropriate diagnosis from the above list of options. Each option may be used once, more than once or not at all.

98. A 40-year-old woman presents with a lump in the left groin. The lump is not reducible and lies below and lateral to the pubic tubercle.
99. A 40-year-old woman who underwent varicose vein surgery recently presents with a lump in the groin. The lump disappears on lying down and transmits cough impulse. It lies just below the groin crease and medial to the femoral pulse.
100. A 60-year-old man presents with a swelling in the groin and the scrotum. Clinical examination reveals a scrotal swelling, and you cannot get above it.
101. A 30-year-old man presents with a reducible groin lump lying above and medial to the pubic tubercle.

Theme: Causes of clubbing

Options

A. Bronchial carcinoma
B. Inflammatory bowel disease
C. Bronchiectasis
D. Liver cirrhosis
E. Subacute bacterial endocarditis
F. Empyema
G. Congenital cyanotic heart disease
H. Cryptogenic fibrosing alveolitis
I. Mesothelioma
J. Lung abscess
K. Familial

Instructions

For each case, choose the single most appropriate diagnosis from the above list of options. Each option may be used once, more than once or not at all.

102. A 39-year-old lawyer presents with rheumatoid arthritis and breathlessness. Her chest radiography shows basal shadows.
103. A retired labourer in a shipbuilding yard presents with worsening dyspnoea and pleuritic pain. His chest radiography shows pleural effusion, and his pulmonary function tests show a restrictive ventilatory defect.
104. A 67-year-old man presents with loss of weight, cough, numbness and tingling in both hands and feet, and muscle weakness.
105. A 58-year-old woman presented with left upper quadrant abdominal pain, which she had had for three weeks. A week before admission, she had developed night sweats, dizziness and confusion. On examination her temperature is 38.7°C, pulse is 120 and blood pressure is 140/60. Abdominal examination showed splenomegaly.
106. A 40-year-old man presents with diarrhoea and lower abdominal discomfort. Also, there is a history of blood and mucus in the stools.
107. A 22-year-old student was noted to be blue and was becoming more short of breath than usual.

Theme: Skin lesions

Options

A. Chicken pox
B. Bullous pemphigoid
C. Pityriasis versicolor
D. Pityriasis rosea
E. Erythema nodosum
F. Stevens–Johnson syndrome

G. Pemphigus vulgaris
H. Erythema marginatum
I. Henoch–Schönlein purpura
J. Erythema multiforme
K. Measles

Instructions

For each skin lesion, choose the single most appropriate diagnosis from the above list of options. Each option may be used once, more than once or not at all.

108. Herald patch: solitary patch with peripheral scaling, most commonly found on the trunk.
109. Target lesions: concentric rings due to a cell-mediated cutaneous lymphocytotoxic response.
110. Thick-walled bullae. Immunofluorescence studies show linear staining of IgG along the basement membrane.
111. Thin walled baullae. Immunoflourescence studies show intercellular staining of IgG within the epidermis.
112. Target lesions with extensive mucous membrane involvement.
113. Umbilicated vesicles, pustules and crusts. Rash distribution is centripetal.
114. Koplik's spots: on the mucosa of the cheeks opposite the molar teeth.

Theme: Operations in gynaecology and their indications

Options

A. Anterior colporrhaphy
B. Marsupialisation
C. Wertheim's hysterectomy
D. Dilatation and curettage
E. Salpingectomy
F. Radical vulvectomy

G. Ventrosuspension
H. Laparoscopy
I. Manchester repair
J. Abdominal tubal ligation
K. Vaginal urethroplasty

Instructions

For each clinical presentation, choose the single most appropriate operation from the above list of options. Each option may be used once, more than once or not at all.

115. Abnormal uterine bleeding, missed abortion or incomplete abortion.
116. Carcinoma of the vulva.
117. Cystourethrocele.
118. Descent of the uterus and laxity of the vaginal walls.
119. Stress incontinence.
120. Blocked Bartholin's duct.

Theme: Urinary problems in women

Options

A. True incontinence
B. Urinary tract infection
C. Overflow incontinence
D. Urge incontinence
E. Frequency of micturition

F. Stress incontinence
G. Urethral syndrome
H. Gonococcal urethritis
I. Urethral prolapse

Instructions

For each sentence below, choose the single most appropriate condition from the above list of options. Each option may be used once, more than once or not at all.

121. Is caused by damage of the urethra during intercourse.
122. Occurs when there is a fistulous communication between the urinary and genital tracts.
123. Occurs when the bladder is full to its limit but is unable to empty.
124. Occurs when there is a sudden increase in intra-abdominal pressure.
125. Occurs when the desire to void is followed almost immediately by voiding.
126. Commonly occurs after catheterisation for urinary incontinence or retention.

Theme: Chest radiography findings in congenital heart diseases

Options

A. Atrial septal defect
B. Coarctation of the aorta
C. L-transposition of the great arteries
D. Fallot's tetralogy
E. D-transposition of the great arteries
F. Patent ductus arteriosus
G. Total anomalous pulmonary venous return
H. Ventricular septal defect
I. Persistent truncus arteriosus
J. Pulmonary stenosis
K. Aortic stenosis

Instructions

For each radiographic finding, choose the single most appropriate diagnosis from the above list of options. Each option may be used once, more than once or not at all.

127. 'Snowman' sign.
128. Egg-shaped heart.
129. Boat-shaped heart.
130. Convex left heart border.
131. '3' sign.
132. Concave main pulmonary artery segment and right aortic arch.

Theme: Paediatric neurological disorders

Options

A. Platybasia
B. Duchenne muscular dystrophy
C. Brain abscess
D. Syringomyelia
E. Glioblastoma multiforme
F. Agenesis of the corpus callosum
G. Arnold–Chiari malformation
H. Cerebral lymphoma
I. Klippel–Feil syndrome
J. Medulloblastoma
K. Tuberous sclerosis

Instructions

For each case, choose the single most appropriate diagnosis from the above list of options. Each option may be used once, more than once or not at all.

133. A 7-month-old infant with infantile spasms and delayed milestones.
134. A 19-year-old student presented with loss of pin-prick and temperature sensation over her shoulders and upper arms. Magnetic resonance imaging (MRI) of the spine showed a fluid-filled cystic cavity in the cervico-thoracic cord.
135. A 3-week-old infant with meningomyelocele presented with progressive head enlargement since birth.
136. A 6-year-old boy presented with clumsiness, abnormal gait and repeated falls. On examination, he had prominent calf muscles and lumbar lordosis. He waddled slightly while walking. Deep tendon reflexes were depressed at the ankles.
137. A previously healthy 5-year-old girl presented with a 3-week history of morning headaches and unsteady gait. CT shows a lesion in the cerebellar vermis.
138. A 9-year-old boy presented with learning difficulties. On examination he is found to have axillary freckles and multiple café au lait spots.

Theme: Causes of syncope

Options

A. Anxiety
B. Munchausen's disease
C. Ménière's disease
D. Epilepsy
E. Orthostatic hypotension
F. Hypoglycaemia

G. Stokes–Adams attack
H. Vasovagal syncope
I. Transient ischaemic attack
J. Carotid sinus syncope
K. Micturition syncope

Instructions

For each case, choose the single most appropriate diagnosis from the above list of options. Each option may be used once, more than once or not at all.

139. A 76-year-old man fell to the floor while standing in a long queue. He regained consciousness within two minutes. He was not incontinent of urine or stools.
140. A 29-year-old secretary had a blackout while working on the computer. She was drowsy for 24 hours after the episode.
141. A 79-year-old woman fell to the floor as she tried to get up from bed. She had recently been started on an angiotensin-converting enzyme (ACE) inhibitor for hypertension.
142. A 55-year-old diabetic collapsed on a long flight. On examination there was pallor and tachycardia.
143. A 71-year-old woman presented with hemiparesis and diplopia which resolved within 24 hours.
144. A 63-year-old man presented following several episodes of loss of consciousness. He usually regained consciousness within a few seconds after falling on the floor. He reported that such episodes were usually preceded by palpitations.

Theme: Autoantibodies

Options

A. Antimicrosomal antibody
B. Cytoplasmic antineutrophil cytoplasmic antibody (C-ANCA)
C. Antidouble-stranded DNA
D. Antiparietal cell antibody
E. Antiacetylcholine receptor antibody
F. Antireticulin antibody
G. Anti-smooth muscle antibody
H. Antistreptolysin
I. Antimitochondrial antibody
J. Perinuclear antineutrophil cytoplasmic antibody
K. Rheumatoid factor

Instructions

For each condition, choose the single most appropriate autoantibody from the above list of options. Each option may be used once, more than once or not at all.

145. Systemic lupus erythematosus.
146. Coeliac disease.
147. Rheumatoid arthritis.
148. Hashimoto's thyroiditis.
149. Myasthenia gravis.
150. Primary biliary cirrhosis.
151. Wegener's granulomatosis.

Theme: Visual field defects

Options

A. Optic chiasmal lesion
B. Frontal lobe lesion
C. Parietal lobe lesion
D. Unilateral occipital lobe lesion
E. Optic nerve lesion
F. Bilateral occipital lobe lesion
G. Ciliary ganglion lesion
H. Temporal lobe lesion
I. Edinger–Westphal nucleus lesion
J. Pretectal nucleus lesion

Instructions

For each visual field defect, choose the single most appropriate anatomical lesion from the above list of options. Each option may be used once, more than once or not at all.

152. Bitemporal hemianopia.
153. Contralateral homonymous hemianopia.
154. Anton's syndrome.
155. Ipsilateral mononuclear field loss.
156. Lower homonymous quadrantanopia.
157. Upper homonymous quadrantanopia.

Theme: Renal calculi

Options

A. Percutaneous nephrolithotomy (PCNL)
B. Extracorporeal shock wave lithotripsy (ESWL)
C. Alkaline diuresis
D. Nephrectomy

E. Percutaneous nephrostomy
F. Expectant management
G. Acid diuresis
H. Intravenous antibiotics
I. Peritoneal dialysis

Instructions

For each case below, choose the single most appropriate management from the above list of options. Each option may be used once, more than once or not at all.

158. A 30-year-old pregnant woman (26 weeks) presents with septicaemia and abdominal pain. Investigations reveal an obstructed right kidney due to a 2 cm calculus. She is commenced on intravenous antibiotics.

159. A 40-year-old man presents with left-side renal colic. Intravenous urography (IVU) shows a 1 cm calculus in the upper third of the ureter. There is no complete obstruction. His symptoms fail to resolve on conservative management.

160. A 20-year-old man presents with renal colic secondary to a 1 cm cystine calculus.

161. A 30-year-old man presents to A&E with a right-side renal colic. IVU shows a 4 mm calculus in the distal part of the ureter with no complete obstruction.

162. A 40-year-old woman is found to have a staghorn calculus in a non-functioning kidney.

163. A 60-year-old man presents with frequent attacks of left-side renal colic due to a 2.5 cm calculus in the renal pelvis. He has a cardiac pacemaker and is known to have a 6 cm aortic aneurysm.

Theme: Malnutrition and malabsorption

Options

A. Scurvy
B. Beri beri
C. Pellagra
D. Riboflavin deficiency
E. Vitamin A deficiency
F. Rickets

G. Vitamin K deficiency
H. Iron deficiency
I. Vitamin B $_{12}$ deficiency
J. Folate deficiency
K. Iodine deficiency

Instructions

For each case, choose the single most appropriate diagnosis from the above list of options. Each option may be used once, more than once or not at all.

164. A 7-year-old boy presenting with night blindness.
165. A 57-year-old alcoholic presenting with peripheral oedema and ascites.
166. A 91-year-old woman presenting with spontaneous bruising and anaemia.
167. A 38-year-old woman presenting with brittle nails and angular stomatitis.
168. A 58-year-old man who had ileal resection for Crohn's disease.
169. A 47-year-old woman with primary biliary cirrhosis presenting with bruising.

Theme: Adverse effects of medications

Options

A. Nifedipine
B. Carbimazole
C. Rifampicin
D. Ampicillin
E. Propranolol
F. Captopril

G. Co-trimoxazole
H. Simvastatin
I. Thiazide diuretic
J. Isoniazid
K. Propyl thiouracil

Instructions

For each case, choose the single most appropriate medication from the above list of options. Each option may be used once, more than once or not at all.

170. A 69-year-old alcoholic was diagnosed to have tuberculosis. He was started on some medications then a few months later developed numbness and tingling in both feet.
171. A 63-year-old diabetic was prescribed a medication for newly diagnosed hypertension. She did not tolerate the medication because of dry persistent cough.
172. A 14-year-old boy presented to his GP with fever, rash and sore throat. The GP diagnosed tonsillitis and started him on an antibiotic. He later developed a blotchy purpuric rash all over his body.
173. A 52-year-old, who had had a triple bypass, complained of myalgia a few weeks after starting a new medication. His liver function tests were abnormal.
174. A 68-year-old was started on a medication for hypertension. He presented later with a tender swollen right first metatarsal joint.
175. A 48-year-old woman with recently diagnosed thyrotoxicosis presented with fever and sore throat.

Theme: Pelvic pain

Options

A. Ectopic pregnancy
B. Ruptured ovarian cyst
C. Pelvic inflammatory disease
D. Appendicitis
E. Endometriosis
F. Inflammatory bowel disease

G. Degenerating fibroid
H. Septic abortion
I. Diverticulitis
J. Septic abortion
K. Ovarian hyperstimulation syndrome

Instructions

For each case, choose the single most appropriate tumour stage from the above list of options. Each option may be used once, more than once or not at all.

176. A 23-year-old woman presents with pelvic pain, fever and vaginal discharge. On examination, there is marked lower abdominal and adnexal tenderness. There is also cervical motion tenderness.
177. A 30-year-old woman presents with primary infertility, pelvic pain, dyspareunia and dysmenorrhoea. On examination, there is beading and tenderness of the uterosacral ligaments and the uterus is fixed and retroverted.
178. A 19-year-old woman presents with severe colicky pain in the right iliac fossa and vomiting. Her periods are regular and pregnancy test is negative. On examination, her temperature is 37.8°C and there is guarding rigidity.
179. A 27-year-old woman is admitted with vaginal bleeding and pelvic pain. She missed her last period and has had early morning sickness over the last week. On examination, her blood pressure is 100/60, pulse is 110 and she is apyrexial.
180. A 35-year-old woman under treatment for infertility presents with pelvic pain, weight gain and abdominal distension. On examination, there is shifting dullness.
181. A 25-year-old woman presents with severe pelvic pain, vaginal bleeding and fever. She has a positive pregnancy test.

Theme: Staging of malignant tumours

Options

A. Endometrial carcinoma: stage IIA

B. Vaginal carcinoma: stage II

C. Endometrial carcinoma: stage IIIA

D. Cervical carcinoma: stage IIA

E. Cervical carcinoma: stage IIIA

F. Endometrial carcinoma: stage IB

G. Ovarian carcinoma: stage IB

H. Cervical carcinoma: stage IIIB

I. Vaginal carcinoma: stage III

J. Vulvar carcinoma: stage II

K. Ovarian carcinoma: stage IIA

Instructions

For each case of malignancy described below, choose the single most appropriate tumour stage from the above list of options. Each option may be used once, more than once or not at all.

182. The carcinoma involves the cervix and upper vagina but has not extended to the lateral pelvic walls or to the lower third of the vagina, and there is no parametrial involvement.
183. The carcinoma involves the endocervical glands as well as the body of the uterus.
184. The carcinoma involves the cervix, pelvic sidewall and hydronephrosis or non-functioning kidney.
185. The carcinoma involves both ovaries with metastases to the uterus and tubes.
186. The carcinoma invades the serosa of the body of the uterus with positive peritoneal cytology.
187. The carcinoma involves the vagina and extends to the pelvic sidewall.

Theme: Pulmonary diseases in children

Options

A. Pulmonary sequestration
B. Asthma
C. Tuberculosis
D. Bronchopulmonary dysplasia
E. Bronchogenic cyst
F. Cystic fibrosis
G. Pulmonary arteriovenous fistula
H. Laryngomalacia
I. Massive pulmonary embolism
J. Tracheo-oesophageal fistula
K. Pulmonary haemosiderosis

Instructions

For each case, choose the single most appropriate diagnosis from the above list of options. Each option may be used once, more than once or not at all.

188. A 4-year-old girl presented with a history of recurrent pneumonia and failure to gain weight. On examination, wheezes and crepitations were heard and her fingers showed clubbing.

189. A 7-week-old infant presents with a 6-week history of noisy breathing. It is inspiratory in nature and increases when the baby is crying or during respiratory infections. It disappears completely when the baby is asleep.

190. A 5-year-old child presents with a history of chronic left lower lobe pneumonitis. On contrast bronchography, the area involved fails to fill, outlined by bronchi that are filled.

191. A 4-year-old child presents with a history of dyspnoea, cyanosis, clubbing, haemoptysis and epistaxis. On examination, there is generalised telangiectasia. Blood tests show polycythaemia.

192. A 1-year-old child presents with a history of coughing, especially with feedings, and recurrent chest infections.

193. A 6-year-old boy presents to A&E with dyspnoea, wheezing and cough. On examination, he is slightly cyanosed. His respiratory rate is 30, blood pressure is 100/60 and pulse is 110.

Theme: Investigating pulmonary diseases in children

Options

A. Barium swallow
B. Pulmonary angiography
C. Chest radiography
D. Contrast bronchography
E. CT of the chest
F. Fibre-optic bronchoscopy

G. Chest ultrasonography
H. ECG
I. Venous cineangiography
J. Sweat test
K. Echocardiography

Instructions

For each indication, choose the single most appropriate investigation from the above list of options. Each option may be used once, more than once or not at all.

194. To guide needle thoracentesis to sample a pleural effusion.
195. To assess an infant with apnoea.
196. To evaluate a child with chronic cough and wheezing.
197. To differentiate a mediastinal mass from a collapsed lung.
198. To rule out pulmonary arteriovenous fistula.
199. To rule out laryngomalacia.

Theme: Adverse effects of medications

Options

A. Metformin
B. Third generation cephalosporin
C. Lamotrigine
D. Bleomycin
E. Amiodarone
F. Tolbutamide
G. Vancomycin
H. Lithium
I. Phenytoin
J. Doxorubicin
K. Digoxin

Instructions

For each case, choose the single most appropriate medication from the above list of options. Each option may be used once, more than once or not at all.

200. A 67-year-old newly diagnosed diabetic was found lying on the floor in his house. On examination he was pale, hypothermic and brady-cardic. The results were: bicarbonate 13 mmol/l, urea 7.7 mmol/l, sodium 136 mmol/l and potassium 5.1 mmol/l.
201. A 35-year-old epileptic complains of impaired balance and blurring of vision. On examination there is nystagmus.
202. A 72-year-old man under treatment for squamous cell carcinoma of the lung becomes progressively short of breath. On examination there are bilateral basal lung crepitations. Chest radiography shows evidence of lung fibrosis.
203. A 76-year-old woman with paroxysmal supraventricular tachycardia presents with impaired vision, cold intolerance and constipation.
204. A 37-year-old man being treated for bipolar disorder presents with polyuria and coarse tremors.
205. A 91-year-old woman presented with severe urinary tract infection. One week after starting treatment, she developed profuse offensive diarrhoea.

Theme: Liver diseases

Options

A. Gilbert's syndrome
B. Chronic active hepatitis
C. Gaucher's disease
D. Galactosaemia
E. Primary biliary cirrhosis
F. Alcoholic liver cirrhosis

G. Wilson's disease
H. Haemochromatosis
I. Cholecystitis
J. Hepatic adenoma
K. Hepatic amoebiasis

Instructions

For each case, choose the single most appropriate diagnosis from the above list of options. Each option may be used once, more than once or not at all.

206. A 37-year-old woman presented with generalised pruritis for six months. On examination she was tanned and there were spider naevi on her chest. The liver was palpable one finger-breadth below the costal margin as well as the tip of the spleen.

207. A 30-year-old woman presented with anorexia, weight loss, lethargy and arthralgia for 3 weeks. On examination she was pale and jaundiced. The liver was palpable two finger-breadths below the costal margin as well as the tip of the spleen. Test results were: ALP 150 U/l, AST 875 U/l, bilirubin 39 μmol/l, albumin 21 g/l, globulin 52 g/l.

208. A 29-year-old woman presented with acute abdominal pain. Her bowels were regular with normal stools. She was taking oral contraceptive pills. On examination there were no features of chronic liver disease. Pulse 120, blood pressure 90/50 and temperature 37.2°C. Her abdomen was tender with guarding. The right hepatic lobe was palpable.

209. A 40-year-old man presents with worsening limb twitches and facial tics. He has been an inpatient in a psychiatric hospital for the last 5 years. His father had a similar history and died in a psychiatric hospital.

210. A 32-year-old man presented with haematemesis and shock. On examination there were multiple surgical scars over both knees, the right hip and the right hypochondrium. His liver was palpable four finger-breadths below the costal margin.

211. A fit 17-year-old man developed a flu-like illness followed 3 days later by abdominal pain, nausea, vomiting and jaundice. All his blood tests were normal apart from increased unconjugated bilirubin.

Theme: Management of endometriosis

Options

A. Danazol therapy
B. Oestrogen replacement therapy
C. Expectant management
D. Methotrexate
E. Conservative endometriosis surgery
F. GnRH agonists

G. Progestogens
H. Cyclic oral contraceptives
I. Non-steroidal anti-inflammatory drugs (NSAIDs)
J. Radical endometriosis surgery

Instructions

For each case, choose the single most appropriate management from the above list of options. Each option may be used once, more than once or not at all.

212. A 27-year-old journalist presents with an established diagnosis of mild endometriosis. She states that she wants to travel for 3 years before considering a pregnancy.

213. A 23-year-old woman presents with a 7-month history of infertility. Diagnostic laparoscopy shows evidence of mild endometriosis with scattered cul-de-sac implants. She has no other infertility factors.

214. A 33-year-old computer programmer presents with a 4-year history of infertility. A laparoscopic diagnosis of moderate endometriosis is made. Scattered endometrial implants in the pelvis, a 1 cm endometrioma on the right ovary and adhesions between the tube and ovary on each side are found.

215. A 37-year-old woman has just undergone radical endometriosis surgery.

216. A 36-year-old woman completed her treatment for endometriosis 6 months ago. During treatment she suffered from bouts of depression, weight gain and metrorrhagia, but there was no dyspareuria. She now complains of amenorrhoea.

217. A 22-year-old single student is diagnosed with mild endometriosis and dysmenorrhoea.

Theme: Investigating amenorrhoea

Options

A. Measurement of serum prolactin levels
B. Laparoscopy
C. Measurement of TSH levels
D. Measurement of gonadotrophin levels
E. Karyotyping
F. Progesterone challenge
G. Measurement of serum testosterone levels
H. Skull radiography
I. Hysteroscopy
J. Intravenous pyelography
K. Measurement of human chorionic gonadotrophin (β-HCG) levels over 24 hours
L. Measurement of β-HCG levels over one week

Instructions

For each case, choose the single most appropriate investigation from the above list of options. Each option may be used once, more than once or not at all.

218. A 22-year-old woman with previously normal menstrual cycles begins to have irregular cycles and anovulation. Serum prolactin levels are elevated.
219. A 23-year-old nulligravida stopped her oral contraceptive pills to conceive. She had a menstrual flow after the last pack of contraceptive pills then was amenorrhoeic for 7 months.
220. A 25-year-old primipara returns 8 months after delivery complaining of amenorrhoea. Her pregnancy terminated with a caesarean section because of abruptio placentae and foetal distress, with estimated blood loss of 1500 ml from a transient coagulation problem.
221. A 27-year-old nulligravida presents with amenorrhoea. Pregnancy test is negative.
222. A 26-year-old woman presents with amenorrhoea for 7 weeks, vaginal spotting and mild right lower quadrant pain. Her periods have always been irregular. On examination, the uterus is of normal size and the right lower quadrant is tender. Her β-HCG level the day before was 1100 mIU/ml.

Theme: Laryngeal carcinoma

Options

A. Total laryngectomy with or without neck dissection
B. Radiotherapy
C. Hemilaryngectomy (vertical)
D. Supraglottic laryngectomy with or without neck dissection (horizontal)
E. Chemotherapy
F. Excision of the vocal cord mucosa
G. Expectant management
H. Radical neck dissection
I. Modified neck dissection
J. Commando procedure

Instructions

For each case, choose the single most appropriate management from the above list of options. Each option may be used once, more than once or not at all.

223. A 50-year-old man presents with a hoarse voice. Clinical examination and investigations reveal a small invasive carcinoma of the right vocal cord. The right vocal cord is paralysed and there is a 4 cm lymph node in the right anterior neck.
224. A 65-year-old man is found to have a T_1 carcinoma of the vocal cord. There is no involvement of the anterior commissure.
225. A 60-year-old woman is found to have carcinoma in situ of the left vocal cord.
226. A 55-year-old woman is found to have a glottic carcinoma involving the anterior commissure.
227. A fit 70-year-old woman with large supraglottic carcinoma.

Theme: Thyrotoxicosis

Options

A. Radioactive iodine
B. Subtotal thyroidectomy
C. Propranolol
D. Carbimazole
E. Potassium iodide
F. Thyroxine

G. Corticosteroids
H. β-Blockers
I. Radiotherapy
J. Total thyroidectomy
K. Total thyroid lobectomy

Instructions

For each case, choose the single most appropriate management from the above list of options. Each option may be used once, more than once or not at all.

228. A 26-year-old pregnant woman is found to have thyrotoxicosis due to Graves' disease during the second trimester of the pregnancy.
229. A 10-year-old girl presents with thyrotoxicosis. A radioisotope scan shows an enlarged thyroid with uniform uptake throughout.
230. A 30-year-old woman is found to have Graves' disease. She remain thyrotoxic after treatment with carbimazole for one year.
231. A 60-year-old woman is found to have a large toxic nodular goitre.
232. A 50-year-old woman presents with thyroid enlargement. Thyroid function tests are normal. The needle biopsy confirms the diagnosis of Hashimoto's thyroiditis.

Theme: Chest radiography findings

Options

A. Chicken pox pneumonia
B. Mitral stenosis
C. Consolidation
D. Fallot's tetralogy
E. Bronchiectasis
F. Longstanding atrial septal defect

G. Asbestosis
H. Sarcoidosis
I. Left ventricular failure
J. Pneumocystis carinii pneumonia
K. Pulmonary embolus

Instructions

For each set of chest radiographic findings, choose the single most appropriate diagnosis from the above list of options. Each option may be used once, more than once or not at all.

233. Multiple calcified nodules mainly in the lower and mid zones. The nodules are less than 3 mm in diameter.
234. Multiple ring shadows at both lower lobes, giving a 'bunches of grapes' appearance with tramline shadowing.
235. Kerley B lines at each base and bilateral pleural effusion, together with hilar shadows.
236. Uniform well defined shadow in the right upper lobe. Air bronchogram is also visible.
237. Double shadow at the right heart border and elevation of the left main bronchus.
238. Cardiomegaly, prominent right atrium, dilated pulmonary arteries and small aortic knuckle.

Theme: Anaemia

Options

A. Pernicious anaemia
B. Glucose-6-phosphate dehydrogenase (G6PD) deficiency
C. Sickle cell anaemia
D. Hereditary spherocytosis
E. Thalassaemia major
F. Anaemia of chronic disease
G. Autoimmune haemolytic anaemia
H. Macrocytic anaemia
I. Paroxysmal nocturnal haemoglobinuria
J. Iron deficiency anaemia
K. Aplastic anaemia

Instructions

For each case of anaemia described below, choose the single most appropriate diagnosis from the above list of options. Each option may be used once, more than once or not at all.

239. A 55-year-old woman with rheumatoid arthritis who is on non-steroidal anti-inflammatory drugs (NSAIDs) and steroids.
240. A 62-year-old male alcoholic with a megaloblastic bone marrow.
241. A 58-year-old woman with Addison's disease and peripheral neuropathy.
242. A 30-year-old man with abdominal pain and distension. Abdominal ultrasonography shows portal vein thrombosis.
243. A 57-year-old man with recently diagnosed lymphoma.
244. A 27-year-old Italian waiter who becomes rapidly jaundiced after a course of ciprofloxacin.

Theme: Haematological diseases in children

Options

A. β-Thalassaemia
B. von Willebrand's disease
C. Paroxysmal nocturnal haemoglobinuria
D. Iron deficiency anaemia
E. β-Thalassaemia
F. Haemophilia A
G. Sickle cell anaemia
H. Glanzmann's thrombasthenia
I. Anaemia of chronic disease
J. Hereditary spherocytosis
K. Microangiopathic haemolytic anaemia

Instructions

For each of the following features, choose the single most appropriate diagnosis from the above list of options. Each option may be used once, more than once or not at all.

245. Decreased haemoglobin, mean corpuscular volume (MCV), mean corpuscular haemoglobin (MCH) and mean corpuscular haemoglobin concentration (MCHC). Increased total iron binding capacity.
246. Reduced synthesis of α-globin chains leading to haemolysis.
247. Normal MCV. Decreased serum iron and total iron binding capacity. Increased serum ferritin.
248. Defect in spectrin.
249. Red blood cells unusually sensitive to the action of haemolytic complement.
250. Prolonged partial thromboplastin time (PTT) and bleeding time. Decreased ristocetin cofactor.

Theme: Paediatric oncology

Options

A. Wilms' tumour
B. Non-Hodgkin lymphoma
C. Osteogenic sarcoma
D. Ewing's tumour
E. Medulloblastoma
F. Acute non-lymphocytic leukaemia
G. Neuroblastoma
H. Histiocytosis X
I. Acute bacterial lymphadenitis
J. Acute lymphoblastic leukaemia
K. Lymphoblastic lymphoma
L. Rhabdomyosarcoma

Instructions

For each case, choose the single most appropriate diagnosis from the above list of options. Each option may be used once, more than once or not at all.

251. A 3-year-old boy presents with a large left-sided abdominal mass. Intravenous urography (IVU) shows a mass within the left kidney which encroaches on the collecting system. Chest radiography shows multiple pulmonary nodules.

252. A 10-year-old boy with diagnosed haemophilia presents with a 4-week history of enlarging left supraclavicular mass. The mass does not regress with factor VIII therapy.

253. A 12-year-old girl presents with a 3-day history of fever and a 3 cm warm, tender and fluctuant right anterior cervical lymph node.

254. An 18-month-old boy presents with periorbital echymoses and a large right loin mass. On examination, he was anaemic and a large right-sided mass distinct from the kidney is palpable. Bone marrow shows clumps of primitive cells. Bone scan shows increased activity in both orbits.

255. A 3-year-old girl presents with a 3-week history of morning headaches, vomiting and unsteady gait. CT shows a lesion in the cerebellar vermis.

256. A 14-year-old boy presents with a 2-week history of pain and swelling in the right thigh. Radiography of the right thigh shows a soft tissue mass with concentric layers of new bone formation. Blood tests reveal leucocytosis and elevated erythrocyte sedimentation rate (ESR).

Theme: ECG findings

Options

A. Right bundle branch block
B. Second-degree block (Wenckebach)
C. Hyperkalaemia
D. Pulmonary embolism
E. Sinus arrhythmia
F. Anterior myocardial infarction

G. Left bundle branch block
H. Wolff–Parkinson–White syndrome
I. Complete heart block
J. First-degree block
K. Second-degree block (Mobitz type II)

Instructions

For each item of ECG findings, choose the single most appropriate diagnosis from the above list of options. Each option may be used once, more than once or not at all.

257. Progressive lengthening of PR interval with one non-conducted beat.
258. Constant PR interval but one P wave is not followed by a QRS complex.
259. One P wave per QRS complex, constant PR interval and progressive beat-to-beat change in RR interval.
260. Dominant R in V_1 and inverted T in the anterior chest leads.
261. Peaked P waves, right axis deviation, inverted T waves in leads V_1 to V_3 and tall R waves in V_1.
262. Dominant R waves in V_1, inverted T waves in leads V_1 to V_3 and deep S waves in V_6.

Theme: Psychiatric disorders

Options

A. Depression
B. Post-traumatic stress disorder
C. Schizophrenia
D. Chronic alcoholism
E. Phobia

F. Anxiety neurosis
G. Mania
H. Obsessional neurosis
I. Depersonalisation
J. Hysteria
K. Paranoid state

Instructions

For each case, choose the single most appropriate diagnosis from the above list of options. Each option may be used once, more than once or not at all.

263. A 23-year-old student presents with insomnia, headaches, sweating, palpitations, chest pains and poor appetite.
264. A 35-year-old single woman presents with weight loss, poor appetite, decreased ability to concentrate and guilt feelings.
265. A 19-year-old female student presents with sudden blindness. Neurological examination reveals no abnormality.
266. A 20-year-old man presents with disinhibition, hyperactivity, increased appetite and grandiosity delusions.
267. A 30-year-old man presents with auditory hallucinations, social withdrawal and delusions of persecution.
268. A 21-year-old man presents with compulsions and rituals, which he resists.

Theme: Endocrine tumours

Options

A. Parathyroid adenoma
B. Multiple endocrine neoplasia (MEN) type I
C. MEN type II
D. Carcinoid syndrome
E. Phaeochromocytoma
F. Medullary thyroid carcinoma

G. Parathyroid hyperplasia
H. Insulinoma
I. Follicular carcinoma of the thyroid
J. Prolactinoma
K. Pituitary adenoma secreting growth hormone

Instructions

For each case, choose the single most appropriate diagnosis from the above list of options. Each option may be used once, more than once or not at all.

269. A 40-year-old man presents with hypertension, palpitations and sweating; 24-hour urinary vanillylmandelic acid (VMA) is elevated. The lesion causing the symptoms is localised using an MIBG scan.
270. A 25-year-old woman presents with hypercalcaemia and bilateral nipple discharge. Serum parathyroid hormone and prolactin are elevated.
271. A 40-year-old man presents with recurrent episodes of flushing, colicky abdominal pain and asthma. Urinary 5-hydroxyindole acetic acid (5HIAA) is elevated.
272. A 45-year-old woman presents with hypercalcaemia and goitre. Investigations reveal elevated serum levels of parathyroid hormone and calcitonin. Past medical history includes a right adrenalectomy 3 years previously.
273. A 61-year-old woman presents with stiff joints, myopathy and constipation. Plain radiographs reveal a right renal calculus and evidence of osteitis fibrosa cystica.

Theme: Jaundice

Options

A. Primary biliary cirrhosis
B. Chronic active hepatitis
C. Carcinoma of the head of the pancreas
D. Sclerosing cholangitis
E. Primary hepatocellular carcinoma
F. Cholangiocarcinoma
G. Gilbert's syndrome
H. Dubin–Johnson syndrome
I. Stones in the common bile duct
J. Rotor's syndrome
K. Hepatitis A

Instructions

For each case, choose the single most appropriate diagnosis from the above list of options. Each option may be used once, more than once or not at all.

274. A 12-year-old boy presents with jaundice after a recent episode of tonsillitis. Serum bilirubin rises further on fasting. Ultrasonography scan and liver biopsy reveal no abnormality.

275. A 27-year-old man presents with jaundice. He also describes a 6-month history of bloody diarrhoea. Haemoglobin is 10 g/dl, bilirubin is 75 µmol/l, and aspartate aminotransferase (AST), alanine aminotransferase (ATL), alkaline transferase (ALP) and gamma-glutamyl transferase (GGT) are all raised. Liver function tests improve with ursodeoxycholic acid administration.

276. A 45-year-old woman presents with painless jaundice 4 weeks after laparoscopic cholecystectomy. Bilirubin is 105 µmol/l, AST is 150 U/l and ALP is 750 U/l.

277. A 69-year-old woman presents with jaundice and backache. Clinical examination shows a mass in the right upper quadrant, acanthosis nigricans and superficial thrombophlebitis.

278. A 49-year-old woman with Sjögren's syndrome presents with jaundice and hepatosplenomegaly. Her urine is dark and serum contains antimitochondrial antibody (titre > 1:64); liver biopsy shows ductal destruction, proliferation and granuloma.

Theme: Causes of confusion

Options

A. Dementia
B. Drug overdose
C. Hypothyroidism
D. Post-ictal
E. Alcohol withdrawal
F. Subdural haemorrhage

G. Meningitis
H. Cerebral malignancy
I. Hypoglycaemia
J. Hyponatraemia
K. Cerebrovascular accident

Instructions

For each case of confusion decribed below, choose the single most appropriate diagnosis from the above list of options. Each option may be used once, more than once or not at all.

279. A 70-year-old woman with tingling and numbness in her fingers, constipation and deafness.
280. A 22-year-old soldier with fever and rash.
281. A 69-year-old man with oat cell carcinoma.
282. A 21-year-old woman with oliguria and subchondral pain.
283. A 20-year-old student who has been on insulin for 13 years.
284. A 79-year-old man unable to give any history. On examination, he is incontinent of urine and stools and is bleeding from the mouth.

Theme: Drug overdose

Options

A. Lithium overdose
B. Aspirin overdose
C. Ethanol overdose
D. Benzodiazepine overdose
E. Tricyclic antidepressant overdose

F. LSD overdose
G. β-Blocker overdose
H. Paracetamol overdose
I. Methanol overdose
J. Amphetamine overdose
K. Digoxin overdose

Instructions

For each case of overdose described below, choose the single most appropriate diagnosis from the above list of options. Each option may be used once, more than once or not at all.

285. A 19-year-old student was admitted to A&E with pyrexia and sweating. Her pulse was 120 and blood pressure was 100/60. She also complained of deafness and tinnitus.
286. A 34-year-old man was admitted to A&E unconscious. His temperature was 37.7°C, pulse was 130 and blood pressure was 90/65. Neurological examination showed bilateral extensor plantars. His pupils were dilated. ECG showed sinus tachycardia and occasional ventricular ectopics.
287. A 69-year-old man presented with drowsiness and confusion. His pulse was 48 and his blood pressure is 98/68. ECG showed first-degree heart block and widening of the QRS complex.
288. A 77-year-old woman presented with nausea, vomiting and diarrhoea. She also complained of blurring of vision and flashes of light. On examination, she was slightly confused and her pulse was slow and irregular.
289. A 37-year-old woman with longstanding psychiatric illness was admitted with polyuria, diarrhoea, vomiting and coarse tremor involving both hands.
290. A 24-year-old waitress developed jaundice, right hypochondrial pain and tenderness, hypoglycaemia and oliguria 2 days after an overdose.

Theme: Causes of haemoptysis

Options

A. Pulmonary infarction
B. Tuberculosis
C. Mitral stenosis
D. Foreign body inhalation
E. Haemorrhagic telangiectasia
F. Bronchogenic carcinoma

G. Pneumonia
H. Bronchiectasis
I. Systemic lupus erythematosus (SLE)
J. Wegener's granulomatosis
K. Polyarteritis nodosa

Instructions

For each case, choose the single most appropriate diagnosis from the above list of options. Each option may be used once, more than once or not at all.

291. A 55-year-old smoker with a long history of recurrent chest infection presents with haemoptysis and greenish sputum. on examination he has clubbing and coarse crepitations over the bases of both lungs.
292. A 69-year-old woman who had a total hip replacement a week ago presents with severe chest pain, shortness of breath and haemoptysis.
293. A 52-year-old diabetic presents with fever, pleuritic pain and rusty-coloured sputum.
294. A 45-year-old bank manager presents with cough, pleuritic chest pain and haemoptysis. This was preceded by rhinitis, recurrent epistaxis and haematuria. Chest radiography shows multiple nodular masses.
295. A 69-year-old smoker presents with cough, haemoptysis and weight loss. On examination, there is clubbing and gynaecomastia.
296. A 72-year-old Asian immigrant presents with cough, haemoptysis, night fever and sweating.

Theme: Human leucocytic antigens

Options

A. Coeliac disease
B. Acute pancreatitis
C. Peptic ulcer
D. Schizophrenia
E. De Quervain's thyroiditis
F. Primary biliary cirrhosis

G. Insulin dependent diabetes mellitus
H. Motor neuron disease
I. Haemochromatosis
J. Hydrocephalus
K. Ankylosing spondylitis

Instructions

For each human leucocytic antigen shown below, choose the single most appropriate association from the above list of options. Each option may be used once, more than once or not at all.

297. HLA-B27.
298. HLA-A28.
299. HLA-DR7.
300. HLA-DR4.
301. HLA-B3.
302. HLA-DR8.

Theme: Therapeutics

Options

A. Oestrogens and progestins
B. Androgens
C. Prostaglandin inhibition
D. Hydrocortisone

E. Methotrexate
F. Progestational agents
G. Danazol
H. Clomiphene citrate

Instructions

For each diagnosis, choose the single most appropriate medication from the above list of options. Each option may be used once, more than once or not at all.

303. Congenital adrenal hyperplasia.
304. Dysmenorrhoea.
305. Dysfunctional uterine bleeding.
306. Isosexual precocious puberty.
307. Anovulation.
308. Choriocarcinoma.

Theme: Amenorrhoea

Options

A. Torsion of an ovarian cyst
B. Hydatidiform mole
C. Threatened abortion
D. Physiological amenorrhoea
E. Ectopic pregnancy
F. Androgen excess amenorrhoea

G. Bleeding corpus luteum
H. Hypogonadotrophic amenorrhoea
I. Eugonadotrophic amenorrhoea
J. Hypergonadotrophic amenorrhoea

Instructions

For each case, choose the single most appropriate diagnosis from the above list of options. Each option may be used once, more than once or not at all.

309. A 28-year-old woman whose last menses were 7 weeks ago presents with acute right lower quadrant pain. Serum β-HCG levels are elevated. Pelvic ultrasonography reveals no sac in the uterus and a 3×3 cm right adnexal mass.

310. A 34-year-old woman whose last menses were 6 weeks ago presents with acute lower left quadrant pain but no vaginal bleeding. Serum β-HCG is appropriate for dates. Pelvic ultrasonography reveals no sac in the uterus and a left 3×4 cm adnexal mass.

311. A 28-year-old woman whose last menses were 7 weeks ago presents with heavy vaginal bleeding and lower left quadrant pain. Serum β-HCG levels are low for dates. Pelvic ultrasonography reveals an intrauterine sac without foetal parts.

312. A 14-year-old adolescent with normal sexual development complains of amenorrhoea for 5 months. Her first menses were 10 months ago, after which she has had 3 menses.

313. A 26-year-old nulligravida had a normal menstrual history until 9 months ago, when she began intensive long-distance running. She has not had a menstrual flow since her first marathon 5 months ago.

314. A 19-year-old woman with well developed secondary sexual characteristics presents with amenorrhoea. She has a vaginal pouch, and karyotyping shows XX chromosomes.

Theme: Chest pain

Options

A. Dissecting aortic aneurysm
B. Dressler's syndrome
C. Boerhaave's syndrome
D. Ventricular aneurysm
E. Pulmonary embolism
F. Kawasaki's syndrome

G. Hypertrophic obstructive cardiomyopathy
H. Pneumothorax
I. Right ventricular infarction
J. Cardiac neurosis
K. Reflux oesophagitis

Instructions

For each case, choose the single most appropriate diagnosis from the above list of options. Each option may be used once, more than once or not at all.

315. A 56-year-old dentist had a successful operation for a fracture of the right neck of the femur. Six days later he complained of dyspnoea at rest and chest pain. ECG showed sinus tachycardia and right axis deviation.

316. A 60-year-old porter collapsed while bending to carry a bag. On admission to A&E he regained consciousness but started to vomit, was sweating profusely and complained of chest pain. Chest radiography showed a widened mediastinum.

317. A 70-year-old man is admitted with severe epigastric pain and sweating. Over the last few weeks he has suffered from chest pain and shortness of breath on moderate exercise. On examination, his jugular venous pressure (JVP) is 10 cm above the sternal angle, pulse is 65/min and blood pressure 115/65, and there is bilateral ankle oedema.

318. A 48-year-old alcoholic is admitted to A&E with severe retrosternal pain and shortness of breath. The pain is constant and radiates to the neck and interscapular region. On examination, his pulse is 120, blood pressure is 90/60 and the left lung base is dull on percussion.

319. A 24-year-old engineer presents with worsening shortness of breath and chest tightness. His father had collapsed and died suddenly when he was 33. On examination, the cardiac apex is double and both fourth heart sound and late systolic murmur are audible at the apex.

320. A 26-year-old man presented with severe chest tightness, which was worse on exercise. He had a strong family history of myocardial infarction. On examination, his temperature was 37.8°C, pulse 90 and blood pressure 130/80; there was normal apex, cervical lymphadenopathy, erythematous buccal cavity and polymorphous rash.

Theme: Cerebrovascular disease

Options

A. Transient ischaemic attack (TIA) involving the carotid system
B. Sagital sinus thrombosis
C. Extradural haemorrhage
D. Lateral medullary syndrome
E. Subarachnoid haemorrhage
F. Subdural haemorrhage
G. Cerebellar haemorrhage
H. Lacunar infarction
I. Hypertensive encephalopathy
J. Pseudobulbar palsy
K. TIA involving the vertebrobasilar system

Instructions

For each case, choose the single most appropriate diagnosis from the above list of options. Each option may be used once, more than once or not at all.

321. A 73-year-old man presents with hemianopia, hemisensory loss, hemiparesis and aphasia of 16 hours duration.
322. A 79-year-old woman presents with hemianopia, hemisensory loss, ataxia, choking, dysarthria and vertigo.
323. A 60-year-old hypertensive and diabetic is admitted with acute dizziness, vomiting and difficulty in moving his right arm and leg. On examination, there is Horner's syndrome on the right side.
324. A 58-year-old man presented to A&E with a severe headache and drowsiness which started suddenly while he was working on the computer. He had vomited once. On examination, he was apyrexial, his pulse was 100 and blood pressure was 160/100.
325. A 72-year-old man was referred by his GP for recurrent headaches and fluctuating level of consciousness. There was no history of direct head trauma.

Theme: Lower limb ischaemia

Options

A. Femoropopliteal bypass
B. Percutaneous balloon angioplasty
C. Femorodistal bypass
D. Intra-arterial tissue plasminogen activator infusion

E. Below knee amputation
F. Fasciotomy
G. Lumbar sympathectomy
H. Aortofemoral bypass
I. Axillofemoral bypass
J. Femorofemoral crossover graft

Instructions

For each case, choose the single most appropriate management from the above list of options. Each option may be used once, more than once or not at all.

326. A 65-year-old man presents with intermittent claudication of the left calf. The claudication distance is 100 m. Angiography demonstrates a 1.5 cm stenosis of the left superficial femoral artery.
327. A 73-year-old diabetic woman presents with critical ischaemia of the right leg. Angiography reveals extensive disease of the superficial femoral, popliteal and tibial arteries. Pulse-generated run-off assessment indicates a good run-off in the posterior tibial artery.
328. A 72-year-old man presents with a 4-hour history of acute ischaemia of the left leg. Clinical examination reveals signs of acute ischaemia with no evidence of gangrene. There is no neurological deficit. An urgent arteriogram reveals a complete occlusion of the distal superficial femoral artery most likely caused by thrombosis.
329. A 57-year-old smoker presents with intermittent claudication of the right calf. The claudication distance is 70 m. Angiography reveals a 12 cm stenosis in the proximal superficial femoral artery.
330. A 21-year-old motorcyclist presents with multiple injuries following a road traffic accident. Clinical examination reveals a critically ischaemic right lower leg. The right dorsalis pulse is feeble. The right calf is tense and swollen. The intracompartmental pressure is 55 mmHg. Angiography shows no discontinuity of the arterial tree.

Theme: Thyroid cancer

Options

A. Total thyroid lobectomy
B. Abletive dose of radioactive iodine
C. External beam radiation
D. Chemotherapy
E. Reassure and repeat fine needle aspiration cytology (FNAC) in 12 months

F. Thyroxine
G. Propranolol
H. Carbimazole
I. Subtotal thyroidectomy
J. Total thyroidectomy and removal of the central group of lymph nodes

Instructions

For each case, choose the single most appropriate management from the above list of options. Each option may be used once, more than once or not at all.

331. A 40-year-old woman presents with a solitary nodule in the right thyroid lobe. FNAC suggests follicular adenoma.
332. A 20-year-old woman presents with a 4 cm solid mass in the left thyroid lobe. FNAC reveals papillary carcinoma.
333. A 15-year-old boy presents with a 1 cm solitary thyroid nodule and diarrhoea. FNAC is reported as malignant. Serum calcitonin is raised.
334. A 30-year-old woman presents with a 2 cm thyroid nodule. FNAC suggests a colloid nodule.
335. A 50-year-old woman presents with a thyroid goitre. A core biopsy reveals evidence of lymphoma.

Theme: Inborn errors of metabolism

Options

A. McArdle's disease
B. Gaucher's disease
C. Fanconi's syndrome
D. Homocystinuria
E. Phenylketonuria
F. Galactosaemia

G. Hartnup disease
H. Cystinosis
I. Niemann–Pick disease
J. Cystinuria
K. Fabry's disease

Instructions

For each case, choose the single most appropriate diagnosis from the above list of options. Each option may be used once, more than once or not at all.

336. Mental retardation and epilepsy. Urine analysis shows phenyl pyruvate.
337. Hepatosplenomegaly, pigmentation of exposed parts and anaemia.
338. Muscle cramps and myoglobinuria after exercise.
339. Hepatosplenomegaly, renal tubular defects, cataract and mental retardation.
340. Mental retardation, downwards subluxation of the lens, recurrent thrombosis.
341. Recurrent urinary stones.

Theme: Neurological disorders

Options

A. Multiple sclerosis
B. Lateral medullary syndrome
C. Sagittal sinus thrombosis
D. Guillain–Barré syndrome
E. Motor neurone disease
F. Arnold–Chiari malformation
G. Normal pressure hydrocephalus

H. Myasthenia gravis
I. Herpes simplex encephalitis
J. Peripheral neuritis
K. Benign intracranial hypertension

Instructions

For each case, choose the single most appropriate diagnosis from the above list of options. Each option may be used once, more than once or not at all.

342. A 35-year-old clerk presents with diplopia and fatigue. Her symptoms are worse towards the evening.
343. A 33-year-old carpenter presents with unsteadiness of gait, incoordination of both arms and oscillopsia on downgaze. Clinical examination demonstrates a low hair line, positive Romberg's test and bilateral extensor plantars.
344. A 40-year-old woman presents with increasing weakness and stiffness of her legs. Three years ago she had a similar episode which lasted a few days and resolved on its own. A year after that she developed diplopia for 2 weeks.
345. A 70-year-old man presents with urinary incontinence and poor muscle coordination. On examination he is slightly confused, but apyrexial and there is no papilloedema. Two years ago he had meningitis which was successfully treated by antibiotics.
346. A previously fit 60-year-old lawyer is admitted to A&E with a 3-day history of progressively bizarre and aggressive behaviour. On examination she is confused and pyrexial. EEG shows abnormal complexes over the temporal lobe.
347. A 58-year-old man presents with progressive clumsiness and difficulty in performing fine tasks with both hands. On examination, there is slight wasting of the intrinsic muscles of both hands, but more on the left. Reflexes and coordination are normal and there is no sensory deficit.

Theme: Renal impairment

Options

A. Medullary sponge kidney
B. Renal tubular acidosis
C. Renal vein thrombosis
D. Acute interstitial nephritis
E. Bartter's syndrome
F. Idiopathic hypercalciuria

G. Diabetic nephropathy
H. Cystinuria
I. Renal artery stenosis
J. Lupus nephritis
K. Minimal change
   glomerulonephritis

Instructions

For each case, choose the single most appropriate diagnosis from the above list of options. Each option may be used once, more than once or not at all.

348. A 19-year-old mechanic was started on flucloxacillin for an infected wound. Blood tests done three days later showed evidence of renal failure. Urine was positive for blood and protein. Abdominal ultrasonography showed normal kidneys with no evidence of obstruction.

349. A 35-year-old woman presented with a blood pressure of 190/110 and impaired renal function. Urine microscopy showed scanty red cells and granular casts. Renal biopsy showed linear IgG on glomerular basement membrane.

350. A 40-year-old man presented with renal colic. He had had several similar episodes in the past which were sometimes associated with passing small stones. Abdominal radiography showed calcified opacities in both kidneys. All blood and urinary tests were normal.

351. A 27-year-old woman presented with renal colic. She was previously fit and had no family history of renal problems. Blood tests were all normal but urinary calcium was elevated.

352. A previously fit 17-year-old porter presented with renal colic. On examination, his left flank was tender. Blood tests were normal. Urine microscopy showed hexagonal crystals. Intravenous pyelography (IVP) showed faintly opaque staghorn calculus in the left renal pelvis.

353. A 66-year-old diabetic woman was investigated for hyperkalaemia. She was on indomethacin and glibenclamide. Blood tests showed evidence of renal impairment, hyperkalaemia and hyperchloraemia.

Theme: Radiological investigations

Options

A. Radioisotope bone scan E. CT scan
B. MRI F. Angiogram
C. Ultrasound scan G. Lumbar puncture
D. Duplex scan H. Spiral CT scan

Instructions

For each item, choose the single most appropriate investigation from the above list of options. Each option may be used once, more than once or not at all.

354. Is useful to assess renal size, identify parenchymal pattern and detect renal stones.
355. Is more sensitive for early space-occupying lesions, especially in the posterior cranial fossa.
356. Is contraindicated in a patient who is suspected to have a space-occupying lesion of the brain.
357. Is of great value in patients with possible pulmonary embolism and co-existing cardiorespiratory disease.
358. Is useful in demonstrating the cause of recurrent TIAs.
359. Is efficient in detecting osteolytic bony metastases.

Theme: Vaginal bleeding

Options

A. Retention of a succenturiate lobe
B. Placenta praevia
C. Uterine rupture
D. Cervical carcinoma
E. Ruptured vasa praevia
F. Cervical laceration

G. Thrombocytopenia
H. Implantation in the lower uterine segment
I. Endometrial carcinoma
J. Atonic uterus
K. Placenta accreta

Instructions

For each case, choose the single most appropriate diagnosis from the above list of options. Each option may be used once, more than once or not at all.

360. Following a spontaneous vaginal delivery, a 22-year-old woman continues to bleed in spite of the use of oxytocin. The uterus appears to contract well but then relaxes with increased bleeding.
361. A 28-year-old woman has just delivered her second baby in two years after an oxytocin-induced labour. She is bleeding heavily despite the use of oxytocics. The uterus is well contracted and there is no evidence of vaginal or cervical tears. The baby weighs 4.5 kg.
362. A 32-year-old woman is still bleeding heavily 6 hours after having delivered twins vaginally.
363. A 40-year-old woman who has had no antenatal care presents at term with heavy vaginal bleeding. Her last pregnancy was 14 years ago. Abdominal ultrasonography shows a foetal heart rate of 150 beats per minute and a fundal placenta.
364. A 32-year-old woman presents in active labour with excessive vaginal bleeding. She has had a previous caesarean section. The foetal heart rate is 65 beats per minute.
365. A 28-year-old woman who is 36 weeks pregnant presents with vaginal bleeding, contractions and a tender abdomen.
366. A 31-year-old woman has delivered with a complete placenta praevia by caesarean section. Two hours later, she is noted to have significant postpartum haemorrhage.

Theme: Management of bleeding

Options

A. Endometrial biopsy
B. Oral contraceptive pills
C. Myomectomy
D. Dilatation and curettage
E. Progestin
F. Oral conjugated oestrogen
G. Non-steroidal anti-inflammatory drugs
H. Hysterectomy
I. Oral iron therapy
J. Hormone replacement therapy
K. Laparoscopy

Instructions

For each case, choose the single most appropriate management from the above list of options. Each option may be used once, more than once or not at all.

367. A 46-year-old woman presents having had a one-year history of menometrorrhagia. On examination she is slightly obese, her uterus is of normal size and her blood pressure is 145/100.

368. A 37-year-old woman presents having had a three-month history of menometrorrhagia. She has been on oral contraceptive pills.

369. A 22-year-old nulligravida presents with bleeding which has continued for 3 weeks, the last 4 days of which were heavy bleeding with clots. Her last menstrual period was 3 months before this bleeding episode. Her haemoglobin is 8.7 g/dl.

370. A 32-year-old woman presents with menorrhagia. Her cycles are regular. On examination she is of average build, her uterus is of normal size and her blood pressure is 145/90.

371. A 29-year-old primipara presents with a uterine mass and menorrhagia. On examination, the uterus is a size appropriate to a 15-weeks gestation and a posterior fundal mass is found.

372. A 52-year-old woman with a known myomatous uterus presents with menometrorrhagia. She reports that her menses occur every 6 weeks and that she has had 5–8 days of intermenstrual spotting over the past four cycles.

Theme: Vascular disease

Options

A. Aortofemoral bypass
B. Percutaneous transluminal angioplasty
C. Axillofemoral bypass
D. Femorofemoral crossover graft

E. Lumbar sympathectomy
F. Ileofemoral bypass
G. Femoropopliteal bypass
H. Femorotibial bypass
I. Fasciotomy
J. Below knee amputation

Instructions

For each case, choose the single most appropriate operation from the above list of options. Each option may be used once, more than once or not at all.

373. A 70-year-old man presents with thigh claudication. Angiography demonstrates atherosclerotic narrowing of the distal aorta and proximal common iliac arteries.
374. An 83-year-old woman (a smoker) presents with left thigh and buttock claudication. Angiography reveals a smooth narrowing (1.5 cm in length) in the left common iliac artery.
375. A 75-year-old man presents with severe right calf claudication. Angiography shows narrowing (10 cm length) of the right distal superficial femoral and popliteal arteries. The right posterior tibial artery has a reasonable run-off.
376. A 78-year-old man with severe emphysema presents with severe claudication of the left thigh and calf. Angiography reveals severe atherosclerosis affecting the left common and external iliac arteries. His past medical history includes previous anterior excision of the rectum and postoperative radiotherapy.

Theme: Skeletal pain

Options

A. Osteosarcoma
B. Ewing's sarcoma
C. Tuberculosis
D. Metastases
E. Multiple myeloma
F. Primary hyperpara-
   thyroidism

G. Osteoporosis
H. Osteomyelitis
I. Osteoarthritis
J. Septic arthritis

Instructions

For each case, choose the single most appropriate diagnosis from the above list of options. Each option may be used once, more than once or not at all.

377. A 70-year-old man presents with backache. Plain radiographs show multiple sclerotic areas in the lumbosacral spine.
378. A 50-year-old woman presents with backache and anaemia. Skeletal survey shows multiple lytic lesions in the skull and spine. Urine contains Bence-Jones proteins.
379. A 15-year-old boy presents with a painful swelling around the left knee. A plain radiograph shows a lytic lesion with sunburst appearance.
380. A 60-year-old woman presents with backache. Plain radiographs reveal osteoporosis, bony cysts and subperiosteal bone resorption.
381. A 70-year-old man with a history of Paget's disease of bone presents with a painful swelling of the femur.

Theme: Breathlessness

Options

A. Extrinsic allergic alveolitis
B. Cystic fibrosis
C. Cryptogenic fibrosing alveolitis
D. Histoplasmosis
E. Churg–Strauss syndrome
F. Pneumothorax
G. Allergic bronchopulmonary aspergillosis
H. Pneumocystis carinii pneumonia
I. Goodpasture's syndrome
J. Acute myocardial infarction
K. Pulmonary embolism

Instructions

For each case, choose the single most appropriate diagnosis from the above list of options. Each option may be used once, more than once or not at all.

382. A 50-year-old man presents with progressive burning pains in the sole of his left foot, bilateral cramps in both calves, and left foot drop. He is a known asthmatic and suffers from recurrent sinusitis. Full blood count shows eosinophilia.

383. A 33-year-old man presented with breathlessness at rest, cough and haemoptysis, all of which he had had for a few days. On examination, he is cyanosed and there are bilateral inspiratory and expiratory wheezes. His peak flow rate is normal. Blood investigations show evidence of renal failure.

384. A 73-year-old man presents with pneumonia which he had had for two weeks and which was resistant to antibiotics. He had had asthmatic bronchitis for more than 50 years. Chest radiography shows consolidation of the right upper zone and the left perihilar consolidation. Blood tests show neutrophilia.

385. A 29-year-old farmer presented with worsening cough, breathlessness and flu-like symptoms, which he had had each winter for 3 years. Chest radiography showed fine miliary shadows. Pulmonary function tests showed evidence of restrictive lung disease.

386. A 33-year-old woman presents with worsening breathlessness and dry cough. On examination there is clubbing, dyspnoea, central cyanosis, fine crepitations over the lung bases and accentuated second heart sound.

387. A 61-year-old woman presents with shortness of breath, chest pain and a single episode of haemoptysis. She had a total hip replacement 10 days ago.

Theme: Renal impairment

Options

A. Renal vein thrombosis
B. Medullary cystic disease
C. Bartter's syndrome
D. Berger's disease
E. Renal tubular acidosis
F. Nephrotic syndrome

G. Alport's syndrome
H. Cystinuria
I. Renal artery stenosis
J. Rhabdomyolysis
K. Fanconi's syndrome

Instructions

For each case, choose the single most appropriate diagnosis from the above list of options. Each option may be used once, more than once or not at all.

388. A 10-year-old boy presents with nocturnal enuresis, easy fatiguability and poor progress at school. On examination he looks short and is normotensive. Blood tests show hypokalaemic hypochloraemic alkalosis.
389. A 62-year-old epileptic was found unconscious at home. Blood tests showed evidence of renal failure. Urine dipstick shows blood +++. Ammonium sulphate test shows coloured supernatant.
390. A 12-year-old girl presents with marked oedema. Blood tests show hypoalbuminaemia. Urine shows heavy proteinuria.
391. A 16-year-old student presented with a 4-month history of urinary frequency. Examination showed no abnormalities, apart from a mild hearing impairment. Blood tests showed evidence of mild renal impairment.
392. A 35-year-old man presented with acute abdominal pain. He had been fit till a month ago when he noticed increasing swelling of both legs, up to his pelvis. On examination there was dullness at the right base with decreased air entry. The rest of the examination was normal, apart from tenderness at the right iliac fossa. His blood tests showed evidence of renal failure.
393. A 40-year-old insurance broker presented with backache and pelvic pain. Radiography of the spine showed osteoporotic changes and medullary calcification of the kidney.

Theme: Investigating infertility

Options

A. Vaginal-wall smear
B. Postcoital test
C. Temperature chart
D. Hysterosalpingography
E. Plasma progesterone

F. Semen analysis
G. Endometrial biopsy
H. Cervical mucus studies
I. Laparoscopy
J. Tubal insufflation

Instructions

For each item, choose the single most appropriate investigation from the above list of options. Each option may be used once, more than once or not at all.

394. Assessment of the quantity and quality of cervical mucus and sperm interaction.
395. Detection of intrauterine malformation and pathology.
396. Detection of endometriosis, swellings or adhesions.
397. Detection of tubal block. May be followed by shoulder pain after the procedure.
398. A fern-like pattern is seen in the preovulatory phase but not in the postovulatory phase.

Theme: Teratogenic infections during pregnancy

Options

A. Coxsackie B virus
B. Varicella zoster virus
C. Cytomegalovirus
D. Herpes simplex virus hominis type 2
E. Toxoplasmosis
F. Mumps

G. Hepatitis A
H. Syphilis
I. Malaria
J. Rubella virus

Instructions

For each item, choose the single most appropriate diagnosis from the above list of options. Each option may be used once, more than once or not at all.

399. Only very rarely leads to congenital infection before 16 weeks' gestation but is known to infect all infants born to women with recent infection.
400. Causes birth defects when a mother is infected with a primary infection as opposed to recurrent infection.
401. Surviving infants may exhibit cardiac malformation, hepatitis, pancreatitis or adrenal necrosis.
402. Surviving infants may suffer from microcephaly, persistent patent ductus arteriosus, pulmonary artery stenosis, atrial septal defect, cataract or microphthalmia.
403. The characteristic triad of abnormalities includes chorioretinitis, microcephaly and cerebral calcifications.
404. Not strictly teratogenic, but infants may suffer from endocardial fibroelastosis, urogenital abnormalities, and ear and eye malformations.

Theme: Thyroid disorders

Options

A. Thyroglossal cyst
B. De Quervain's thyroiditis
C. Hypothyroidism
D. Multiple endocrine
   neoplasia (MEN) type I
E. Simple goitre

F. Hashimoto's thyroiditis
G. Graves' disease
H. MEN type II
I. Papillary carcinoma
J. Lymphoma
K. Follicular carcinoma

Instructions

For each case, choose the single most appropriate diagnosis from the above list of options. Each option may be used once, more than once or not at all.

405. A 27-year-old woman presents with fever, sore throat and dysphagia. On examination she has a fine tremor and a diffusely tender thyroid. Radioisotope scan shows no uptake.
406. A 43-year-old woman presents with weight loss despite a good appetite, constipation, frontal headaches and metrorrhagia. She also complains of recurrent dyspepsia and peptic ulcers. Her abdominal radiography shows abdominal stones.
407. A 30-year-old woman presents with weight gain, constipation, lethargy and a flaky rash.
408. A 37-year-old woman presents with weight loss, muscle weakness, oligomenorrhoea, diarrhoea and blurring of vision. On examination, there is exophthalmos and proximal myopathy.
409. A 19-year-old student presents with a neck swelling. On examination, the swelling moves up with swallowing and protrusion of the tongue.
410. A 49-year-old woman presents with goitre. On examination, the thyroid is firm and rubbery. Thyroid microsomal antibodies are positive in high titre.

Theme: Infections

Options

A. Tuberculosis
B. Lyme disease
C. Toxic shock syndrome
D. Salmonellosis
E. Trichinosis
F. Bacillary dysentry

G. Leptospirosis (Weil's disease)
H. Toxoplasmosis
I. Amoebic hepatitis
J. Visceral leishmaniasis
K. Actinomycosis

Instructions

For each case, choose the single most appropriate diagnosis from the above list of options. Each option may be used once, more than once or not at all.

411. A 30-year-old HIV-positive man developed fits. On examination there were generalised lymphadenopathy, tender nodules on his legs, right homonymous hemianopia and mild right pyramidal weakness. CT showed a right frontoparietal space-occupying lesion.

412. A 29-year-old photographer presented with diplopia. He had had a past history of facial palsy and recurrent knee swelling. On examination there was mild meningism and partial left III palsy. There was no evidence of residual VII palsy. Both knees were swollen and tender. There were increased protein and white blood cells in the cerebrospinal fluid.

413. A 19-year-old student presented with acute diplopia, fever and tongue pain. He had had an episode of gastroenteritis during a trip to Alaska 2 weeks earlier. On examination his conjunctivae were swollen and there was bilateral ophthalmoplegia. Tongue movements were weak bilaterally. The rest of the examination was normal.

414. A 42-year-old Asian immigrant presented with a 2-month history of fever and weight loss. On examination there was generalised lymphadenopathy, hepatomegaly and huge splenomegaly. His ankles were swollen but there was no evidence of chronic liver disease.

415. A 27-year-old abattoir worker presented with myalgia and jaundice. On examination his conjunctivae were injected and there was diffuse petechial rash. There was no organomegaly.

416. A 23-year-old woman was admitted with diarrhoea, fever and headache. She was menstruating for 3 days prior to admission. On examination, she is confused and flushed and there is a macular rash and bilateral conjunctivitis. Her pulse is 120 and her blood pressure is 100/65.

Theme: Investigating gastrointestinal disorders

Options

A. Oesophageal manometry
B. Barium swallow
C. Chest radiography
D. Upper gastrointestinal endoscopy and biopsy
E. CT of the chest
F. Motility studies

G. MRI of the abdomen and pelvis
H. CT of the abdomen and pelvis
I. Colonoscopy
J. Barium enema
K. Oesophageal pH testing

Instructions

For each case, choose the single most appropriate investigation from the above list of options. Each option may be used once, more than once or not at all.

417. A 70-year-old alcoholic and heavy smoker presents with a 3-month history of progressive dysphagia and weight loss.
418. A 53-year-old man underwent upper gastrointestinal endoscopy for assessment of dysphagia. Three hours later, he complained of severe chest pain. On examination, there was crepitus in the neck.
419. A 69-year-old man has been on medications for a gastric ulcer for 12 weeks. A repeat upper gastrointestinal series (gastrografin) shows moderate shrinkage of the ulcer.
420. A 57-year-old man with an 8-week history of dysphagia undergoes a barium swallow. It shows a bird's beak deformity of the distal oesophagus with proximal dilatation.
421. A 60-year-old presents with a 2-day history of worsening left lower quadrant abdominal pain. On examination, he is pyrexial and there is tenderness in the left lower quadrant. Full blood count shows leucocytosis.

Theme: Management of myasthenia gravis

Options

A. Corticosteroids
B. Radiotherapy and chemotherapy
C. Partial thymectomy
D. Thymectomy and radiotherapy
E. Thymectomy
F. Expectant management
G. Anticholinesterases
H. Azathioprine
I. Radiotherapy
J. Chemotherapy

Instructions

For each case, choose the single most appropriate management from the above list of options. Each option may be used once, more than once or not at all.

422. Maligant thymoma.
423. Generalised myasthenia gravis with a benign thymoma.
424. Ocular myasthenia gravis with a normal thymus gland.
425. Benign thymoma.
426. Generalised myasthenia gravis with a normal thymus gland.

Theme: Rheumatology

Options

A. Scleroderma
B. Giant cell arteritis
C. Ankylosing spondylitis
D. Polymyositis
E. CREST syndrome
F. Systemic lupus erythematosus

G. Polyarteritis nodosa
H. Rheumatoid arthritis
I. Reiter's syndrome
J. Antiphospholipid syndrome
K. Sjögren's syndrome

Instructions

For each case, choose the single most appropriate diagnosis from the above list of options. Each option may be used once, more than once or not at all.

427. A 38-year-old man presented with progressive breathlessness, unproductive cough and difficulty in swallowing. He also noted that his hands become painful and pale in cold weather. Chest radiographs showed patchy shadows in both mid-zones and bases. Radiography of the hands showed calcification.

428. A 31-year-old travel agent presents with painful knees, red eyes and dysuria. He has just returned from a trip to Spain.

429. A 78-year-old woman presented with headache, anorexia and fever which she has had for a few weeks. Erythrocyte sedimentation rate (ESR), C-reactive protein (CRP) and platelets were elevated; haemoglobin was low.

430. A 36-year-old woman complains of recurrent chest pain, which is worse on inspiration, and progressive breathlessness. She also suffers from Raynaud's phenomenon. On examination she has a butterfly rash, and a pericardial rub is audible.

431. A 45-year-old woman presented with a 4-month history of multiple joint pain and progressive difficulty climbing stairs. Muscle biopsy was normal. EMG showed spontaneous fibrillation, high frequency repetitive potentials and polyphasic potentials on voluntary contractions.

432. A 46-year-old woman complains of dryness of the mouth and eyes, joint pain and difficulty in swallowing. Schirmer tear test and Rose Bengal staining are both positive.

Theme: Sexually transmitted diseases

Options

A. Syphilis
B. Gonorrhoea
C. AIDS
D. Lymphogranuloma venereum
E. Granuloma inguinale
F. Molluscum contagiosum
G. Herpes simplex hominis virus type 2
H. Gardnerella vaginalis
I. Chlamydia trachomatis
J. Trichomoniasis
K. Candidiasis

Instructions

For each case, choose the single most appropriate diagnosis from the above list of options. Each option may be used once, more than once or not at all.

433. A 23-year-old man presents with dysuria, urethral discharge and joint pain. Gram staining shows Gram-negative intracellular diplococci.

434. A 27-year-old African immigrant presents with painful fixed inguinal lymphadenopathy. Three weeks earlier he had had a painless papule on his genitalia which ulcerated, then healed.

435. A 31-year-old woman presents with fever, myalgia, headache and multiple painful shallow ulcers in the vulva. On examination, there are also ulcers in the cervix and tender inguinal lymphadenopathy. Four weeks after treatment and recovery her symptoms recur but are less severe.

436. A 37-year-old multipara presented with vaginal discharge. Ten days earlier she had used a medication for yeast infection. She also complains of a strong odour after intercourse.

437. A 20-year-old married woman presents with a 2-week history of sporadic lower abdominal, accompanied by a low grade fever. She also reports an increasing amount of cloudy, non-irritating discharge and dysuria.

438. A 25-year-old sexually active woman presents with mucopurulent vaginal discharge, pelvic pain and fever. The symptoms begin towards the end of her menstrual period.

Theme: Adverse effects of medications

Options

A. Danazol
B. Clomifene citrate
C. Methotrexate
D. GnRH analogues
E. Oxytocin
F. Bromocriptine

G. Progestogens
H. Hormone replacement therapy
I. Prednisolone
J. Non-steroidal anti-inflammatory drugs

Instructions

For each set of adverse effects, choose the single most appropriate causative medication from the above list of options. Each option may be used once, more than once or not at all.

439. Weight gain, acne, growth of facial hair, voice changes, decreased breast size, atrophic vaginitis and dyspareunia.
440. Osteoporosis in cases of prolonged use, hot flushes, decreased libido and vaginal dryness.
441. Breakthrough bleeding, weight gain, depression, prolonged amenorrhoea after starting treatment.
442. Visual disturbances, ovarian hyperstimulation, hot flushes, headache, weight gain, depression and abdominal discomfort.
443. May increase the risk of breast cancer and deep venous thrombosis. Side-effects include weight gain, abdominal discomfort, depression and jaundice.
444. Headache, postural hypotension and Raynaud's phenomenon. High doses may cause retroperitoneal fibrosis.

Theme: Anaesthesia during labour

Options

A. Spinal anaesthesia
B. Epidural anaesthesia
C. General anaesthesia
D. Pudendal block
E. Paracervical block

F. Intravenous meperidine
G. Intramuscular morphine
H. Naloxone
I. Butorphanol

Instructions

For each case, choose the single most appropriate method of anaesthesia from the above list of options. Each option may be used once, more than once or not at all.

445. A 28-year-old woman is in labour. The vertex is on the perineum and the infant's head is visible at the perineum with each push. She has had no analgesia or anaesthesia up to this point.

446. A 26-year-old woman presents with painful uterine contractions occurring every 3 minutes. On examination, she is dilated 2 cm and @60% effaced. Three hours later, she still has the same contraction pattern but her cervix is still only 2 cm dilated.

447. A 25-year-old woman presents with painful uterine contractions occurring every 2 minutes. She is dilated 3 cm with the vertex at 1 station. Two hours later she is 6 cm dilated with the vertex at +1 station.

448. A 30-year-old woman is in labour. Her cervix is 4 cm dilated. Five minutes after being given anaesthesia, she is in respiratory arrest.

449. A 22-year-old woman is in labour. Her cervix is 2 cm dilated and she has regular contractions occurring every 3 minutes. She is allergic to meperidine. Ten minutes after being given anaesthesia, the foetal heart rate drops to 50 beats per minute.

Theme: Malabsorption

Options

A. Chronic pancreatitis
B. Crohn's disease
C. Cystic fibrosis
D. Intestinal lymphangiectasia
E. Immunodeficiency
F. Pancreatic carcinoma

G. Coeliac disease
H. Whipple's disease
I. Thyrotoxicosis
J. Postinfectious malabsorption
K. Obstructive jaundice

Instructions

For each case, choose the single most appropriate diagnosis from the above list of options. Each option may be used once, more than once or not at all.

450. A 38-year-old man presented with recurrent arthritis, diarrhoea and steatorrhoea. On examination, there were bilateral small knee effusions. Small bowel biopsy showed periodic acid–Schiff (PAS)-positive material in the lamina propria.
451. A 50-year-old architect presented with a 1-year history of lethargy, weight loss, diarrhoea and low back pain. On examination, there was evidence of proximal myopathy and mild pitting oedema. Faecal fat excretion was increased.
452. A 65-year-old man presents with severe epigastric pain and weight loss. The pain is severe and radiating to the back. On examination, there is a palpable epigastric mass and hepatomegaly.
453. A 38-year-old man presents with bloody diarrhoea, abdominal discomfort and weight loss. On examination, there is a tender palpable mass in the right iliac fossa.
454. A 19-year-old student presents with abdominal pain and diarrhoea. She has had recurrent chest infections for most of her life.
455. A 58-year-old alcoholic complains of epigastric pain of 5 months' duration. The pain gets worse after heavy alcohol consumption. He also complains of diarrhoea and weight loss. Abdominal radiography shows multiple calcifications.

Theme: Congenital cardiac lesions

Options

A. Atrial septal defect
B. Ebstein's anomaly
C. Congenital pulmonary stenosis
D. Ventricular septal defect
E. Patent ductus arteriosus
F. Hypertrophic obstructive cardiomyopathy
G. Fallot's tetralogy
H. Coarctation of the aorta and bicuspid aortic valve
I. Dextrocardia
J. Transposition of the great arteries
K. Congenital aortic stenosis

Instructions

For each case, choose the single most appropriate diagnosis from the above list of options. Each option may be used once, more than once or not at all.

456. A 27-year-old woman presented with headache. On examination, her blood pressure was 165/115, pulse was 90, and there was an ejection click in the aortic area and an ejection systolic murmur all over the precordium and back.

457. A 39-year-old man presented with progressive breathlessness and palpitations. On examination, the JVP was elevated with a prominent 'a' wave and there was a pulmonary ejection systolic murmur. ECG showed a right bundle branch block with large P waves.

458. A 12-year-old boy with a history of recurrent chest infections presented with worsening shortness of breath. On examination there was systolic thrill at the left lower sternal edge, pansystolic murmur and accentuated second heart sound.

459. A 21-year-old man presented with worsening shortness of breath. He had been told that he had had a murmur since he was a child. On examination there was a continuous murmur and the pulse was bounding.

460. A 5-year-old boy was referred for poor growth and worsening shortness of breath. On examination, he was cyanosed and there was clubbing. There was an ejection systolic murmur, single second heart sound and a parasternal heave. Chest radiography showed right ventricular hypertrophy and a small pulmonary artery.

461. An infant was referred for heart failure and cyanosis. On examination there was elevated JVP, hepatomegaly, pansystolic murmur at the lower left sternal edge and third heart sound. Chest radiography showed a large globular heart. ECG showed right bundle branch block.

Theme: Management of gastrointestinal disorders

Options

A. CT of the abdomen
B. Oesophageal manometry
C. Motility studies
D. Mesenteric angiography
E. Percutaneous transhepatic cholangiogram
F. Barium enema

G. Upper gastrointestinal endoscopy
H. Barium meal
I. Ultrasound scan
J. Erect and supine abdominal radiography

Instructions

For each case, choose the single most appropriate investigation from the above list of options. Each option may be used once, more than once or not at all.

462. A 49-year-old alcoholic presents with haematemesis and melaena. He is stable after being transfused 2 units of blood.
463. A 56-year-old man presents with massive persistent fresh rectal bleeding. A recent barium enema showed no evidence of diverticulosis or tumours. Nasogastric suction showed yellow bile and no evidence of bleeding.
464. A 59-year-old man presents with a 2-day history of worsening crampy abdominal pain, constipation and recurrent vomiting. On examination, his abdomen is distended, with high-pitched bowel sounds. There is no localised tenderness or rectal mass.
465. A 65-year-old woman presents with a one-year history of pain in the right upper quadrant exacerbated by eating rich foods.
466. A 68-year-old man presents with obstructive jaundice and severe weight loss of 2 months' duration. Abdominal ultrasonography shows a 5 cm mass with dilated bile ducts in the head of the pancreas.

Theme: Blood supply to the brain

Options

A. Basilar artery
B. Anterior cerebral artery
C. Superior cerebellar artery
D. Posterior cerebral artery
E. Anterior communicating artery
F. Middle cerebral artery
G. Circle of Willis

H. Posterior communicating artery
I. Anterior inferior cerebellar artery
J. Anterior spinal artery
K. Posterior inferior cerebellar artery

Instructions

For each area of the brain, choose the single most appropriate blood supply from the above list of options. Each option may be used once, more than once or not at all.

467. Broca's area of speech.
468. Trigeminal nerve nucleus in the medulla oblongata.
469. Visual cortex.
470. Leg area in the motor cortex.
471. Anterior aspect of the pons.
472. Arm and face areas in the motor cortex.

Theme: Chest pain in pregnancy

Options

A. Aortic dissection
B. Massive pulmonary embolism
C. Pulmonary infarction
D. Myocardial infarction
E. Aortic rupture

F. Hysteria
G. Pneumothorax
H. Oesophageal spasm
I. Pericarditis
J. Musculoskeletal pain

Instructions

For each case, choose the single most appropriate diagnosis from the above list of options. Each option may be used once, more than once or not at all.

473. A 30-year-old pregnant woman (31 weeks) presents with severe chest pain of acute onset. There is a family history of ischaemic heart disease. Clinical examination demonstrates dyspnoea, cyanosis, hypotension (90/50) and distended neck veins.
474. A 24-year-old pregnant woman (27 weeks) presents with a 6-hour history of pleuritic chest pain and haemoptysis. She has a family history of ischaemic heart disease.
475. A tall slim 30-year-old pregnant woman (26 weeks) presents with central chest pain, hypotension (90/40) and tachycardia. There is a family history of ischaemic heart disease.
476. A 33-year-old pregnant woman (29 weeks) presents with inspiratory chest pain. The pain is much less when she sits up and leans forward. She had an upper respiratory tract infection a week earlier.

Theme: Blood film

Options

A. Infectious mononucleosis
B. Iron deficiency anaemia
C. Malaria
D. Thrombotic thrombocytopenic purpura
E. Megaloblastic anaemia
F. Sickle cell disease

G. Multiple myeloma
H. Acute myeloid leukaemia
I. Myelofibrosis
J. β-Thalassaemia major
K. Chronic lymphatic leukaemia

Instructions

For each blood film, choose the single most appropriate diagnosis from the above list of options. Each option may be used once, more than once or not at all.

477. Hypochromic microcytic red cells and cigar-shaped cells.
478. Poikilocytosis, anisocytosis, macrocytosis, tear drop cells and hyper-segmented polymorphs. The macrocytes are oval rather than round.
479. Microcytosis, anisocytosis, poikilocytosis, hypochromia, target cells and tear drop cells.
480. Sickle cells, target cells and nucleated red cells.
481. Leucoerythroblastic blood film with immature white cells and nucleated red cells, anisocytosis, poikilocytosis and tear drop cells.
482. Stacking of red cells into rouleaux and abnormal plasma cells.

Theme: Arthritis

Options

A. Systemic lupus
   erythematosus
B. Antiphospholipid syndrome
C. Reiter's disease
D. Rheumatoid arthritis
E. Felty's syndrome

F. Giant cell arteritis
G. Sjögren's syndrome
H. Scleroderma
I. Polyarteritis nodosa
J. Osteoarthritis
K. Pseudogout

Instructions

For each case, choose the single most appropriate diagnosis from the above list of options. Each option may be used once, more than once or not at all.

483. A 53-year-old woman complains of redness, swelling and stiffness in the distal interphalangeal joints of her hands, but has no other joint complaints.
484. A 60-year-old previously fit man presented with a 2-month history of fatigue, dyspnoea on exertion, abdominal pain and progressive numbness in his feet. He recently developed mild polyarthritis in his hands. On examination, there was evidence of left median nerve mononeuritis. Chest radiography showed cardiomegaly.
485. A 79-year-old man complains of pain and swelling of the right knee. He has bilaterally swollen wrists, metacarpophalangeal (MCP), proximal interphalangeal (PIP) and distal phalangeal (DIP) joints. His knee is also swollen with limitation of range of motion by pain. Radiography shows calcification of the meniscal cartilage of the knee.
486. A 22-year-old woman presents with a 3-week history of fever, pleuritic chest pain, stiffness and swelling in the wrists, MCP joints and PIP joints. On examination, there is bilateral pretibial oedema.
487. A 27-year-old man presented with low back pain, pain in the right knee and sore eyes. His past history included an episode of diarrhoea 3 weeks earlier, and he had a positive family history of back pain. Pelvic radiography showed sclerosis and erosion of the lower joint margins.
488. A 77-year-old woman with long-standing rheumatoid arthritis presented with fever and dysuria. Her past history included recurrent chest and urinary infections. On examination, she was hyperpigmented and emaciated. Her hands and feet were severely deformed. Abdominal examination revealed splenomegaly but no hepatomegaly or lymphadenopathy.

Theme: Electrolyte imbalance

Options

A. Hyperparathyroidism
B. Addison's disease
C. Hyperthyroidism
D. Oat cell carcinoma
E. Cushing's disease
F. Diabetes mellitus

G. Diabetes insipidus
H. Pyloric stenosis
I. Psychogenic polydipsia
J. Multiple myeloma
K. Vitamin D deficiency

Instructions

For each biochemical profile, choose the single most appropriate diagnosis from the above list of options. Each option may be used once, more than once or not at all.

489. Hyponatraemia, hyperkalaemia, hypoglycaemia and increased urea.
490. Hyponatraemia, hypokalaemia and metabolic alkalosis.
491. Hypernatraemia, hypokalaemia and hyperglycaemia.
492. Hypoalbuminaemia, hypercalcaemia and hyperuricaemia.
493. Hyponatraemia, hypokalaemia and hypercalcaemia.
494. Hypercalcaemia, hypophosphataemia and increased alkaline phosphatase.

Theme: Dermatomes

Options

A. C8

B. T7

C. L4

D. S3

E. T1

F. L5

G. T10

H. C2

I. S1

J. L5

K. C4

Instructions

For each dermatome, choose the single most appropriate nerve root from the above list of options. Each option may be used once, more than once or not at all.

495. The big toe and the anteromedial aspect of the leg.
496. The little finger and the medial aspect of the palm and dorsum of the hand.
497. The little toe and the posterolateral aspect of the heel.
498. A transverse band crossing the umbilicus.
499. The medial aspect of the arm and forearm.
500. The middle three toes and the lateral aspect of the front of the leg.

Theme: Cranial nerves

Options

A. I	**G.** VII
B. II	**H.** VIII
C. III	**I.** IX
D. IV	**J.** X
E. V	**K.** XI
F. VI	**L.** XII

Instructions

For each nerve supply, choose the single most appropriate cranial nerve from the above list of options. Each option may be used once, more than once or not at all.

501. Motor fibres to the trapezius and sternomastoid.
502. Motor fibres to the muscles of the tongue.
503. Sensory fibres to the tonsillar fossa and pharynx plus taste fibres to the posterior third of the tongue.
504. Motor fibres to the muscles of mastication.
505. Motor fibres to the superior oblique muscle.
506. Motor fibres to the lateral rectus muscle.

Theme: Clinical features of AIDS

Options

A. Painful feet
B. Acute hemiparesis
C. Acute focal neurology and seizures
D. Progressive visual impairment
E. Progressive leg weakness
F. Acute delirium
G. Proximal muscle weakness
H. Fasciculation
I. Progressive hemiparesis
J. Impotence

Instructions

For each diagnosis, choose the single most appropriate clinical feature from the above list of options. Each option may be used once, more than once or not at all.

507. Cryptococcal meningitis.
508. Non-bacterial thrombotic endocarditis.
509. Chronic inflammatory demyelinating polyneuropathy.
510. Central nervous system lymphoma.
511. Chronic sensory polyneuropathy.
512. Cerebral toxoplasmosis.

Theme: Physical signs of cardiac lesions

Options

A. Aortic regurgitation
B. Hypertrophic obstructive cardiomyopathy
C. Patent ductus arteriosus
D. Aortic stenosis
E. Atrial septal defect
F. Tricuspid regurgitation
G. Mitral regurgitation
H. Coarctation of the aorta
I. Mitral stenosis
J. Ventricular septal defect
K. Transposition of the great arteries

Instructions

For each physical sign, choose the single most appropriate diagnosis from the above list of options. Each option may be used once, more than once or not at all.

513. Pulsatile liver.
514. Positive Hill's sign.
515. Third heart sound.
516. Soft, single second heart sound.
517. Loud first heart sound.
518. Cardiac apex double in character.

Theme: Haematological diseases

Options

A. Paroxysmal nocturnal haemoglobinuria
B. Thrombotic thrombocytopenic purpura
C. Protein C deficiency
D. Sickle cell anaemia
E. Antiphospholipid syndrome
F. Disseminated intravascular coagulopathy
G. Polycythaemia rubra vera
H. Trousseau's syndrome
I. Waldenström's macroglobulinaemia
J. Multiple myeloma
K. Myelofibrosis

Instructions

For each case, choose the single most appropriate diagnosis from the above list of options. Each option may be used once, more than once or not at all.

519. A 65-year-old woman with mitral stenosis presented with painful red lesions on her left leg and chest, 4 days after starting warfarin.
520. A 62-year-old man presents with symptoms of deep venous thrombosis in the left leg and the right forearm. One month ago, he was treated by warfarin for deep venous thrombosis of the right leg.
521. A 29-year-old woman presented with deep venous thrombosis of the left calf. She had a history of recurrent abortions and arthritis.
522. A 42-year-old man presented with portal vein thrombosis. He had a 4-year history of chronic iron deficiency anaemia with unknown source of blood loss.
523. A 31-year-old woman presented with vaginal bleeding 6 days after an abortion. Two hours after admission, she started fitting then lapsed into a coma. On examination, her temperature was 38.3°C and pulse was 160. Blood tests showed anaemia, thrombocytopenia and a normal clotting profile. Renal function was markedly impaired.
524. A 75-year-old woman presented with headache, visual floaters, weight loss, lethargy and recurrent epistaxis. On examination, she was pale with generalised lymphadenopathy and hepatosplenomegaly. Fundal examination showed right retinal vein thrombosis.

Theme: Diarrhoea

Options

A. Viral gastroenteritis
B. Ulcerative colitis
C. Coeliac disease
D. Laxative abuse
E. Thyrotoxicosis
F. Campylobacter infection

G. Pseudomembranous colitis
H. Giardia lamblia infestation
I. Collagenous colitis
J. Irritable bowel syndrome
K. Chronic pancreatitis

Instructions

For each case, choose the single most appropriate diagnosis from the above list of options. Each option may be used once, more than once or not at all.

525. A 52-year-old woman presented with a 4-year history of recurrent non-bloody diarrhoea. All investigations were normal (including radiography and endoscopy) apart from elevated ESR and colonic biopsy which showed an eosinophilic band in the subepithelial layer.
526. A previously fit 22-year-old man presented with acute bloody diarrhoea, crampy abdominal pain and low grade fever. His symptoms resolved spontaneously in 6 days and never recurred.
527. A 28-year-old woman presented with chronic watery diarrhoea. The stools showed a positive osmotic gap. Her diarrhoea stopped within 3 days after admission and fasting.
528. A previously healthy 21-year-old man presented with a 6-week history of bloody diarrhoea, crampy abdominal pain and fever. Proctosigmoidoscopy showed bleeding and friable colonic mucosa.
529. A 27-year-old woman developed severe water diarrhoea 12 days after starting antibiotics for pelvic inflammatory disease. Proctosigmoidoscopy showed plaque-like lesions.
530. An anxious 28-year-old sales assistant presented with a 4-month history of diarrhoea alternating with constipation. The stools were usually soft and there was no history of bleeding. No abnormality was found on examination. All investigations, including flexible fibre-sigmoidoscopy and radiography, were normal.

Theme: Thyroid function tests

Options

A. Non-toxic goitre
B. Hashimoto's thyroiditis
C. Subacute thyroiditis
D. Anaplastic carcinoma
E. Nephrotic syndrome
F. Pregnancy
G. Hypothyroidism
H. Thyroid binding globulin deficiency
I. Riedel's thyroiditis
J. Graves' disease

Instructions

For each biochemical profile, choose the single most appropriate diagnosis from the above list of options. Each option may be used once, more than once or not at all.

531. Elevated serum T_4 and increased radioactive iodine uptake.
532. Elevated serum T_4 and low radioactive iodine uptake.
533. Elevated serum T_4 and low T_3 resin uptake.
534. Decreased serum T_4 and low T_3 resin uptake.
535. Normal serum T_3 and T_4 in a patient with a neck mass.
536. Normal serum TSH, free T_4 and T_3. Decreased serum total T_4.

Theme: Rheumatology

Options

A. Rheumatoid arthritis
B. Scleroderma
C. Reiter's syndrome
D. Sjögren's syndrome
E. Dermatomyositis
F. Systemic lupus erythematosus

G. Polymyalgia rheumatica
H. Polymyositis
I. Giant cell arteritis
J. Takayasu's arteritis
K. Churg–Strauss syndrome
L. Antiphospholipid syndrome

Instructions

For each case, choose the single most appropriate diagnosis from the above list of options. Each option may be used once, more than once or not at all.

537. A 52-year-old woman complains of a 4-month history of Raynaud's phenomenon, progressive skin tightness, thickening of the fingers and hands, dyspnoea on exertion and dysphagia.
538. A 22-year-old woman complains of loss of appetite, low-grade fever, shoulder and buttock pains, and severe cramps in her arms and hands during exercise. On examination, her pulse is weak in both arms, her blood pressure is 75/55 in the left arm, 60/40 in the right arm and 125/75 in both legs.
539. A 52-year-old man complains of a gritty sensation in his eyes and dry mouth. He also complains of arthralgias in both hands and knees. On examination, there are multiple purpuric lesions over both calves and ankles.
540. A 32-year-old man presents with a rash on his penis, pain in the left heel and right-sided stiffness in the lower back upon arising in the morning. Two weeks earlier, he had had an episode of diarrhoea.
541. A 73-year-old man presents with persistent malaise, anorexia, pain in the shoulders and hips, and loss of 10 kg over the last 10 weeks. On examination, there is mild painful limitation of hip and shoulder motion and muscle tenderness but no weakness.
542. A 25-year-old woman presents with deep venous thrombosis in the right leg. Her past history includes three miscarriages. Her blood tests show mild thrombocytopenia and a positive serology test for syphilis.

Theme: Physical signs of congenital heart diseases

Options

A. Patent ductus arteriosus
B. Atrial septal defect
C. Aortic stenosis
D. Ebstein's anomaly
E. Ventricular septal defect
F. Pulmonary stenosis
G. Coarctation of the aorta

H. Fallot's tetralogy
I. L-transposition of the great arteries
J. Eisenmenger's syndrome
K. D-transposition of the great arteries

Instructions

For each of the following physical findings, choose the single most appropriate diagnosis from the above list of options. Each option may be used once, more than once or not at all.

543. Continuous murmur.
544. Absent femoral pulses.
545. Fixed, widely split second heart sound.
546. Harsh pansystolic murmur best heard at the lower left sternal border.
547. Wide splitting of the first and second heart sounds.
548. Right ventricular heave, single second heart sound and a harsh systolic ejection murmur along the sternal border.

Theme: Management of thoracic disorders

Options

A. Chest tube insertion
B. Pericardiocentesis
C. Ventilation/perfusion scan
D. Lung function tests
E. CT of the chest
F. Echocardiography

G. MRI of the chest
H. Thoracotomy and decortication
I. Local wound exploration
J. Antibiotics

Instructions

For each case, choose the single most appropriate management from the above list of options. Each option may be used once, more than once or not at all.

549. A 42-year-old man is brought to A&E with a stab wound to the right chest in the third intercostal space in the anterior axillary line. He is hypotensive and complains of shortness of breath. On examination, breath sounds are absent on the right side of the chest.

550. A 57-year-old man is brought to A&E after a road traffic accident. He is conscious and stable but has severe bruising of the anterior chest. His chest radiograph shows widened mediastinum and a small left pleural effusion.

551. A 67-year-old alcoholic presents with a 2-week history of fever and purulent expectoration. Chest radiography shows an air–fluid level in the upper lobe of his left lung.

552. A 60-year-old smoker presents with haemoptysis. His chest radiograph shows a 2 cm non-calcified lesion of the upper lobe of the left lung. A radiograph taken 4 years earlier was normal.

Theme: Renal pathology

Options

A. Wegener's granulomatosis
B. Goodpasture's syndrome
C. Lupus nephritis
D. Multiple myeloma
E. Diabetic nephropathy
F. Berger's disease

G. Toxaemia of pregnancy
H. Polycystic kidneys
I. Chronic interstitial nephritis
J. Renal papillary necrosis
K. Medullary sponge kidney

Instructions

For each renal pathology, choose the single most appropriate diagnosis from the above list of options. Each option may be used once, more than once or not at all.

553. Necrotising granulomatous vasculitis.
554. Nodular glomerulosclerosis.
555. Positive congo red staining with amyloid.
556. Positive fluorescent antinuclear antibody (ANA).
557. Glomerular capillary endotheliosis.
558. Highly cellular crescentic proliferative glomerulonephritis.

Theme: Tumour markers

Options

A. Calcitonin
B. HCG (human chorionic gonadotrophin)
C. CA 15-3
D. Thyroglobulin
E. CA 125
F. CEA (carcinoembryonic antigen)

G. CA 19-9
H. PSA (prostate-specific antigen)
I. S-100
J. AFP (α-fetoprotein)

Instructions

For each tumour, choose the single most appropriate tumour marker from the above list of options. Each option may be used once, more than once or not at all.

559. Carcinoma of the head of the pancreas.
560. Ovarian carcinoma.
561. Breast carcinoma.
562. Prostatic carcinoma.
563. Hepatocellular carcinoma.

Theme: Tumour markers

Options

A. CA 15-3
B. CA 125
C. CA 19-9
D. CEA (carcinoembryonic antigen)
E. AFP (α-fetoprotein)
F. HCG (human chorionic gonadotrophin)
G. Calcitonin
H. Thyroglobulin
I. PSA (prostate-specific antigen)
J. S-100

Instructions

For each tumour, choose the single most appropriate tumour marker from the above list of options. Each option may be used once, more than once or not at all.

564. Medullary thyroid carcinoma.
565. Hepatocellular carcinoma.
566. Rectal carcinoma.
567. Papillary thyroid carcinoma.
568. Maligant melanoma.

Theme: Neurological disorders

Options

A. Guillain–Barré syndrome
B. Labyrinthitis
C. Anterior spinal artery occlusion
D. Alzheimer's disease
E. Shy–Drager syndrome
F. Multiple sclerosis

G. Glioblastoma multiforme
H. Vertebral artery dissection
I. Chronic inflammatory demyelinating polyneuropathy
J. Cauda equina syndrome
K. Parkinson's disease
L. Meningioma

Instructions

For each case, choose the single most appropriate diagnosis from the above list of options. Each option may be used once, more than once or not at all.

569. A 24-year-old diver developed headache, dizziness, right hemiparesis and loss of pain and temperature sensation in the right facial and left side of the body following a dive.
570. A healthy 76-year-old woman presented after a fall. On examination, there was weakness of both legs with loss of pain and temperature sensation and areflexia. Her bladder was distended.
571. A 58-year-old man presented with a 10-month history of impotence. On examination, there were bradykinesia, rigidity, postural hypotension, ataxia and tremors.
572. A 75-year-old woman presented with a 3-week history of headache and progressive confusion. On examination, she had right hemianopia. CT showed a large irregularly enhancing mass in the left parietal lobe. There was no evidence of systemic disease.
573. A healthy 72-year-old woman presented with auditory hallucinations. During the interview she seemed incoherent. Examination was unremarkable.
574. A 73-year-old man presented with a 3-month history of progressive difficulty walking. On examination, he had distal weakness in the arms and legs. Muscle stretch reflexes were absent. Motor nerve conduction velocities were slowed.

Theme: Vasculitis

Options

A. Microscopic polyangiitis
B. Takayasu's arteritis
C. Wegener's granulomatosis
D. Kawasaki's disease
E. Henoch–Schönlein purpura
F. Churg–Strauss syndrome

G. Polyarteritis nodosa
H. Giant cell arteritis
I. Cryoglobulinaemic vasculitis
J. Goodpasture's syndrome
K. Behçet's disease

Instructions

For each case, choose the single most appropriate diagnosis from the above list of options. Each option may be used once, more than once or not at all.

575. A 22-year-old woman presented with worsening headache, nausea, painful neck and fever. A year ago she had developed pain in her legs on running. On examination, her blood pressure was 190/105, femoral pulses were weak with a radiofemoral delay, and an abdominal bruit was heard.

576. A 16-year-old student presented with severe chest pain. On examination, his temperature was 38.8°C, blood pressure was 100/60 and pulse was 120. There was also conjunctival congestion, polymorphous rash and palpable lymphadenopathy.

577. A 79-year-old man presented with acute loss of vision in his left eye which he had had for 24 hours. He had had severe temporal headaches for about 6 months. On examination, the left optic disc was swollen with flame-shaped haemorrhage at 7 o'clock. Eye movements were full and painless.

578. A 28-year-old man presented with fever, myalgia and abdominal pain. On examination, his temperature was 38.8°C, blood pressure was 190/110 and pulse was 120. His abdomen was tender with guarding and absent bowel sounds.

579. A 42-year-old man presented with shortness of breath and sinusitis. He also complained of numbness and weakness of the left leg, which he had had for 3 months. On examination, his temperature was 38.1°C and there was evidence of left sensory motor neuropathy. Full blood count showed eosinophilia. Chest radiography showed pulmonary infiltrates.

580. A 13-year-old boy was admitted with a tender swollen left knee and a tender right elbow. His past history included recurrent sore throats

and dull abdominal pain for a few days. On examination, his temperature was 37.9°C and there was some periumbilical tenderness. Both urine and stools were positive for blood.

Theme: Acute abdominal pain

Options

A. Acute intermittent porphyria
B. Acute pancreatitis
C. Ischaemic colitis
D. Sigmoid volvulus
E. Intussusception
F. Familial Mediterranean fever
G. Acute appendicitis
H. Paroxysmal nocturnal haemoglobinuria
I. Diverticulitis
J. Meckel's diverticulitis
K. Perforated peptic ulcer
L. Inflammatory bowel disease

Instructions

For each case, choose the single most appropriate diagnosis from the above list of options. Each option may be used once, more than once or not at all.

581. A 63-year-old man presented with vomiting, bloody diarrhoea and acute pain in the left iliac fossa. He had had a similar episode which followed a heavy meal and he had had two myocardial infarcts over the last 10 years. On examination, his temperature was 37.7°C and his left iliac fossa was tender with no guarding.

582. A 72-year-old woman presented with sudden severe left-sided abdominal pain while straining to pass stools. She had had a long history of constipation. On examination, she was afebrile. Her abdomen was distended, particularly on the left, and tender and tympanitic with increased bowel sounds.

583. A 24-year-old Cypriot student presented with severe abdominal pain, fever and a tender swollen left knee. Four weeks ago he had also suffered from a similar swelling in his right ankle. On examination, his temperature was 39.0°C and his abdomen was diffusely tender. Urinalysis showed protein +++, blood negative and glucose negative.

584. A 34-year-old Spanish lawyer presented with severe colicky central abdominal pain radiating to the back. She had recently been started on barbiturates for convulsions and insomnia. On examination, her temperature was 38.1°C and there was a laparotomy scar with no evidence of organomegaly.

585. A 37-year-old woman presented with worsening fatigue and intermittent abdominal pain. Three weeks ago, she had had an axillary vein thrombosis. On examination, she was mildly jaundiced. Full blood count showed anaemia, leucopenia and thrombocytopenia. Urine analysis was positive for blood.

586. A 13-year-old girl presented with a 6-hour history of pain in the right iliac fossa and fresh bleeding per rectum. On examination, her temperature was 36.5°C, blood pressure was 100/60 and pulse was 120. Oral mucosa was normal. Abdomen was soft, with no organomegaly. All investigations were normal, including a full blood count, clotting profile, urea and electrolytes, gastroscopy and sigmoidoscopy.

Theme: Risk factors for malignancies

Options

A. Asbestosis
B. Aniline dye
C. Hypercalcaemia
D. Pernicious anaemia
E. Early menarche and late menopause

F. Epstein–Barr virus
G. Nulliparity
H. Ulcerative colitis
I. Multiple sexual partners
J. Xeroderma pigmentosum
K. Polycystic kidney disease

Instructions

For each malignant tumour, choose the single most appropriate risk factor from the above list of options. Each option may be used once, more than once or not at all.

587. Gastric carcinoma.
588. Ovarian carcinoma.
589. Colorectal carcinoma.
590. Bladder carcinoma.
591. Lung carcinoma.
592. Burkitt's lymphoma.

Theme: Haematuria

Options

A. Urinary tract infection
B. Transitional cell carcinoma of the ureter
C. Renal adenocarcinoma
D. Ureteric calculus
E. Prostatic carcinoma
F. Prostatic hyperplasia

G. Urinary bladder calculus
H. Haemorrhagic cystitis
I. Glomerulonephritis
J. Polycystic disease of the kidney
K. Vasculitis

Instructions

For each case, choose the single most appropriate diagnosis from the above list of options. Each option may be used once, more than once or not at all.

593. A 51-year-old man presents with a 2-month history of haematuria and pain in the right flank. Urine microscopy confirms haematuria (Hb 19 g/dl, WCC 1300/mm$_3$, haematocrit 59%).
594. A 20-year-old woman presents with urinary frequency, haematuria and lower abdominal pain.
595. A 75-year-old man presents with haematuria and backache. Plain radiographs show sclerotic areas in the lumbosacral spine.
596. A 46-year-old worker in the rubber industry presents with haematuria and renal colic. A plain abdominal radiograph shows no abnormality.
597. A 35-year-old surgeon presents with severe flank pain, nausea and vomiting. Urine microscopy shows red blood cells and crystals (Hb 14 g/dl, WCC 1500/mm^3).

Theme: Genetic disorders

Options

A. Turner's syndrome
B. Triple X syndrome
C. Fragile X syndrome
D. Down's syndrome

E. Patau's syndrome
F. Klinefelter's syndrome
G. Double Y syndrome
H. Edwards' syndrome

Instructions

For each set of clinical findings, choose the single most appropriate diagnosis from the above list of options. Each option may be used once, more than once or not at all.

598. Low-set ears, micrognathia, rocker-bottom feet and learning difficulties.
599. Low-set ears, cleft lip, micro-ophthalmia and learning difficulties.
600. Tall, fertile male, minor mental and psychiatric illness.
601. Infertile male, testicular atrophy, gynaecomastia and learning difficulties.
602. Flat face, slanting eyes, simian crease, hypotonia and learning difficulties.
603. Primary amenorrhoea, short stature, cubitus vulgus and normal IQ.

Theme: Metabolic disturbances

Options

A. Hypokalaemia
B. Hyponatraemia
C. Hypervitaminosis A
D. Hyperkalaemia
E. Hypoglycaemia
F. Hyperglycaemia

G. Hypocalcaemia
H. Hypermagnesaemia
I. Hypernatraemia
J. Hypercalcaemia
K. Hypophosphataemia

Instructions

For each clinical presentation, choose the single most appropriate metabolic disorder from the above list of options. Each option may be used once, more than once or not at all.

604. Restlessness, confusion, irritability, seizures and coma.
605. Muscle weakness, bradycardia and hypotension. ECG shows tall peaked T waves.
606. Sweating, palpitations, tremors, drowsiness and fatigue.
607. Muscle weakness and ectopic beats. ECG shows flattened or inverted T waves.
608. Perioral paraesthesia, carpopedal spasm and generalised seizures.
609. Severe abdominal pain, nausea, vomiting, constipation, polyuria and polydipsia.

Theme: Erythropoietin level

Options

A. Polycythaemia secondary to hepatoma
B. Congenital spherocytosis
C. Polycythaemia rubra vera
D. Thalassaemia minor
E. Anaemia of chronic disease

F. Renal failure
G. Aplastic anaemia
H. G6PD (glucose-6-phosphate dehydrogenase) deficiency
I. von Willebrand's disease
J. Haemophilia A

Instructions

For each biochemical profile, choose the single most appropriate diagnosis from the above list of options. Each option may be used once, more than once or not at all.

610. Normal or slightly elevated plasma erythropoietin with a variable response to exogenous erythropoietin.
611. Elevated plasma erythropoietin with a poor response to exogenous erythropoietin.
612. Extremely high plasma erythropoietin levels.
613. Low or absent plasma erythropoietin.
614. Low erythropoietin levels with a good response to exogenous erythropoietin.

Theme: Immunodeficiency disorders

Options

A. DiGeorge syndrome
B. Nezelof syndrome
C. Wiskott–Aldrich syndrome
D. Leucocyte adhesion deficiency
E. Ataxia telangiectasia
F. Severe combined immunodeficiency (SCID)
G. Bruton's agammaglobulinaemia
H. Chédiak–Steinbrinck–Higashi syndrome
I. Chronic granulomatous disease
J. Job syndrome
K. Selective IgA deficiency

Instructions

For each assay below, choose the single most appropriate diagnosis from the above list of options. Each option may be used once, more than once or not at all.

615. Low lymphocytic count.
616. Increased IgE and eosinophilia.
617. Giant lysosomal granules in granulocytes.
618. Low serum calcium level.
619. Nitroblue tetrazolium test (NBT)
620. Abnormal platelet number and morphology.

Theme: Investigations during pregnancy

Options

A. Kleihauer–Betke test
B. Bile acids and liver function test
C. Oral glucose tolerance test
D. Amniocentesis
E. Full blood count
F. Abdominal ultrasound
G. 24-hour urine protein excretion

H. Sickling test
I. Skin allergy test
J. ECG
K. Maternal DNA sampling
L. Urine for microscopy, culture and sensitivity

Instructions

For each case, choose the single most appropriate investigation from the above list of options. Each option may be used once, more than once or not at all.

621. A 36-year-old para 3+1 has a triple test which showed that her baby has an increased risk of having Down's syndrome.
622. A 24-year-old primiparous woman presents at 33 weeks' gestation with itching.
623. A 23-year-old primiparous woman presents at 31 weeks' gestation with profuse vaginal bleeding. She is Rhesus negative.
624. A 32-year-old para 2+1 presents at 36 weeks' gestation with a blood pressure of 175/100 and proteinuria ++.
625. A 30-year-old primiparous 35-weeks pregnant woman is noted to have a symphyseal-fundal height of 28 cm.

Theme: Bone profile interpretation

Options

A. Hypoparathyroidism
B. Pseudohypoparathyroidism
C. Pseudopseudohypopara-
   thyroidism
D. Primary
   hyperparathyroidism
E. Tertiary
   hyperparathyroidism
F. Chronic renal failure

G. Sarcoidosis
H. Di George's syndrome
I. Paget's disease of bone
J. Bone metastases
K. Osteomalacia
L. Multiple myeloma

Instructions

For each case, choose the single most appropriate diagnosis from the above list of options. Each option may be used once, more than once or not at all.

626. A 19-year-old man presents to A&E with an epileptic fit. He is noted to have a short stature and small hands. X-ray of hands shows short fourth and fifth metacarpals. Investigations: normal renal function and glucose; Ca 1.72 mmol/l, phosphate 2.12 mmol/l and albumin 40 g/l.

627. A 47-year-old vegan presents to her GP with ache in both legs and hips. Investigations: normal full blood count, renal function and thyroid function tests; Ca 2.15 mmol/l, phosphate 0.95 mmol/l, alkaline phosphatase 480 iu/l and albumin 31 g/l.

628. A 63-year-old man presents to his GP with a 3-month history of low back pain. Investigations: Hb 8.9 g/dl, MCV 84 fl, WCC 6.7×10^9/l, platelets 251×10^9/l, ESR 96 mm in first hour, Ca 2.88 mmol/l, alkaline phosphatase 128 iu/l and albumin 30 g/l.

629. A 9-year-old girl is brought to A&E after a grand mal fit. X-ray shows normal hand bones. Investigations: normal renal function and glucose. Ca 1.69 mmol/l, phosphate 1.93 mmol/l, alkaline phosphatase 162 iu/l and albumin 38 g/l.

630. A 62-year-old woman presents to her GP with increasing tiredness, thirst, polyuria and recurrent epigastric pain. Normal full blood count, glucose and ESR. Urea 10.9 mmol/l, creatinine 135 mmol/l, Ca 3.28 mmol/l, phosphate 0.69 mmol/l, alkaline phosphatase 172 iu/l and albumin 39 g/l.

Theme: Amenorrhoea

Options

A. Thyrotoxicosis
B. Hypothyroidism
C. Prolactinoma
D. Pregnancy
E. Menopause
F. Primary ovarian failure

G. Hypogonadal hypogonadism
H. Polycystic ovarian syndrome
I. Cryptomenorrhoea
J. Turner's syndrome
K. Bulimia nervosa
L. Anorexia nervosa

Instructions

For each case, choose the single most appropriate diagnosis from the above list of options. Each option may be used once, more than once or not at all.

631. A 17-year-old woman presents with a three-month history of secondary amenorrhoea. She admits to binge-eating and is concerned about being overweight. She goes to the gym daily and her BMI is 15.4.
632. A 37-year-old woman presents with a four-month history of secondary amenorrhoea, and weight loss of 7 kg despite a good appetite. Pregnancy test is negative.
633. An 18-year-old woman presents with a six-month history of secondary amenorrhoea, hirsutism and weight gain of 4 kg. She has suffered from irregular periods since menarche at the age of 13. Her BMI is 31.
634. A 17-year-old virgin with normal secondary sexual characteristics presents to her GP with primary amenorrhoea. O/E: a bluish bulge is seen just inside the hymen and the uterus shows 12 weeks' gestation.
635. A 42-year-old woman presents with a four-month history of secondary amenorrhoea, recurrent headaches and reduced visual acuity. On further questioning, she admits to occasional staining of her bra with milk.

Theme: Abdominal pain

Options

A. Perforated duodenal ulcer
B. Perforated diverticular disease
C. Gastritis
D. Small bowel obstruction
E. Large bowel obstruction
F. Diverticulitis

G. Gastric ulcer
H. Duodenal ulcer
I. Acute septic peritonitis
J. Acute appendicitis
K. Ischaemic colitis
L. Ulcerative colitis

Instructions

For each case, choose the single most appropriate diagnosis from the above list of options. Each option may be used once, more than once or not at all.

636. An 81-year-old woman presents with a four-day history of recurrent lower abdominal pain, distension and absolute constipation. O/E: distended abdomen which is soft and non-tender on palpation. Percussion is hyperresonant.

637. A 52-year-old man presents with a six-hour history of severe persistent epigastric pain. O/E: he appears very distressed, with pain, blood pressure is 110/60, pulse is 120 bpm, his abdomen is very tender particularly at the epigastrium, with guarding rigidity. Bowel sounds are absent.

638. A 47-year-old man presents with a four-day history of worsening periumbilical colicky pain, vomiting and abdominal distension. He last opened his bowels two days ago. His past medical history is unremarkable apart from a hernia surgery which was performed two years ago.

639. A 79-year-old woman with a long history of constipation presents with a five-day history of worsening left iliac fossa pain and feeling generally unwell. O/E: temperature is 37.6°C, tender left iliac fossa with guarding rigidity.

640. A 78-year-old heavy smoker with a history of diabetes mellitus, hypertension and ischaemic heart disease presents with a five-day history of left iliac fossa pain and bloody diarrhoea. Stool cultures are negative. Colonoscopy shows an ulcer at the rectum.

Theme: Rectal bleeding

Options

A. Ulcerative colitis
B. Crohn's disease
C. Infective colitis
D. Ischaemic colitis
E. Anal fissure
F. Haemorrhoids

G. Bleeding disorder
H. Clotting disorder
I. Diverticular disease
J. Anal carcinoma
K. Colonic carcinoma
L. Colonic polyp

Instructions

For each case, choose the single most appropriate diagnosis from the above list of options. Each option may be used once, more than once or not at all.

641. A 24-year-old man presents with a ten-day history of bloody diarrhoea and abdominal cramp-like pain. Flexible sigmoidoscopy shows diffuse mucosal erythema. Biopsy shows oedema and inflammatory changes. Stool culture grows *E. coli*.

642. A 23-year-old woman presents with a four-month history of bloody diarrhoea, abdominal pain and weight loss of 7 kg. O/E: swollen lips, buccal ulcers and raised red tender lesions on the shins. Colonoscopy shows multiple rectal ulcers with a normal mucosa in between.

643. A 30-year-old woman presents with a three-month history of bloody diarrhoea and colicky abdominal pain. Colonoscopy shows diffuse mucosal erythema throughout the rectum and descending colon. Stool cultures are negative.

644. A 72-year-old man presents with a two-month history of intermittent rectal bleeding, constipation and weight loss of 5 kg. Plain abdominal x-ray and proctoscopy are normal. Full blood count shows microcytic anaemia.

645. A 33-year-old man presents with a two-month history of occasional painless bright rectal bleeding lining the stools and also on tissue paper. Full blood count is normal.

Theme: Eye drops

Options

A. Timolol
B. Pilocarpine
C. Azelastine
D. Guanethidine
E. Tropicamide
F. Phenylephrine

G. Atropine
H. Fluorescein
I. Carbachol
J. Hypromellose
K. Dipivefrine
L. Apraclonidine

Instructions

For each case, choose the single most appropriate eye drops from the above list of options. Each option may be used once, more than once or not at all.

646. A 68-year-old type II diabetic man arrives for his annual follow-up at the diabetes clinic. A mydriatic is needed for funduscopy.
647. A 21-year-old man is referred to the ophthalmology clinic with a four-year history of congested eyes and lacrimation occurring every spring, lasting for about two months.
648. A 71-year-old man under treatment for non-Hodgkin's lymphoma presents with a two-day history of severe left ocular pain and photophobia. O/E: the left eye is very congested and multiple small vesicles are noted at the nose.
649. A fit and healthy 69-year-old woman visits her optician to change her reading glasses. Funduscopy shows cupping of the optic disc.
650. A 49-year-old woman is referred to the rheumatology clinic with a four-month history of itchy eyes, dry mouth and bilateral parotid enlargement. Schirmer's test is positive.

Theme: Urinary symptoms in children

Options

A. Henoch-Schönlein purpura
B. Bacterial cystitis
C. Renal vein thrombosis
D. Acute pyelonephritis
E. Vesicoureteric reflux
F. Haemolytic-uraemic syndrome
G. Nephroblastoma

H. Acute glomerulonephritis
I. Congenital polycystic kidneys
J. Benign recurrent haematuria
K. Horseshoe kidney
L. Renal TB

Instructions

For each case, choose the single most appropriate diagnosis from the above list of options. Each option may be used once, more than once or not at all.

651. A 4-year-old girl presents with dysuria, frequency of micturition and itching in the pubic region.
652. A 5-year-old girl presents with oliguria, haematuria and diffuse oedema. She had a sore throat three weeks earlier.
653. A 7-year-old boy with a history of recurrent painless haematuria is fully investigated and all his results are normal (including IVU and abdominal ultrasound scan).
654. A 1-year-old boy presents with fever and marked abdominal distension. Urinalysis shows microscopic haematuria. There is no family history of any renal disease.
655. A 12-year-old boy presents with acute abdominal pain. He has a three-month history of bilateral knee pain. O/E: skin rash mainly in his lower limbs; urinalysis shows microscopic haematuria.

Theme: Viral infections in children

Options

A. Rotavirus
B. Hepatitis B virus
C. Molluscum contagiosum
D. Cytomegalovirus
E. Epstein Barr virus
F. Rubella virus

G. Mumps virus
H. Influenza virus
I. Parainfluenza virus
J. Polio virus
K. Coxsackie virus
L. Measles virus

Instructions

For each case, choose the single most appropriate viral infection from the above list of options. Each option may be used once, more than once or not at all.

656. A 4-year-old child develops papular lesions with umbilicated centres on his trunk. They disappear within seven months. The child remains well throughout.
657. A 6-month-old baby presents with fever, cough and tachypnoea. Chest x-ray shows bilateral widespread shadows. His mother is HIV positive.
658. The 2-year-old son of Albanian refugees presents with fever, increased salivation and swollen left cheek.
659. A 2-year-old boy presents with a 12-hour history of fever, cough and hoarseness of voice. While waiting in A&E, he develops stridor.
660. A 5-year-old child develops severe diarrhoea, nausea and vomiting one day after returning from a school trip.

Theme: Haematemesis

Options

A. Erosive gastritis
B. Oesophageal carcinoma
C. Oesophageal varices
D. Peptic ulcer
E. Mallory-Weiss tear
F. Gastric leiomyoma

G. Hiatus hernia
H. Oesophagitis
I. Gastric carcinoma
J. Zollinger-Ellison syndrome
K. Bleeding disorder
L. Clotting disorder

Instructions

For each case, choose the single most appropriate diagnosis from the above list of options. Each option may be used once, more than once or not at all.

661. A 25-year-old painter presents early on a Sunday morning with vomiting of fresh blood. He admits to drinking nine pints of beer on Saturday night. He had vomited several times before finally vomiting about 40 cc of fresh blood.

662. A 76-year-old woman is admitted to ITU with extensive burns and hypotension. She is resuscitated but within 24 hours she vomits 200 cc of coffee-ground fluid.

663. A 69-year-old heavy smoker presents with recurrent coffee-ground vomiting and weight loss of 14 kg over the last three months. He also admits to loss of appetite, epigastric discomfort and sensation of fullness after small meals.

664. A 54-year-old Egyptian farmer with a history of schistosomiasis presents with haematemesis and melaena. O/E: palpable hepatosplenomegaly and caput medusae.

665. A 42-year-old woman with a history of recurrent peptic ulcers, which didn't respond in the past to ranitidine, presents with coffee-ground vomiting. Endoscopy shows multiple duodenal ulcers. Abdominal CT scan shows a small pancreatic mass.

Theme: Methods of contraception

Options

A. Periodic abstinence
B. Condom
C. Intrauterine contraceptive device
D. Combined oral contraceptive pill
E. Coitus interruptus

F. Sterilisation
G. Vaginal diaphragm
H. Cervical cap
I. Depot progesterone
J. Progesterone-only pills
K. Spermicide
L. Mifepristone

Instructions

For each statement, choose the single most appropriate method of contraception from the above list of options. Each option may be used once, more than once or not at all.

666. Is contraindicated in migraine or a history of deep venous thrombosis.
667. Is the most common method of contraception in the UK for females aged between 35 and 45.
668. Is only suitable in a stable relationship.
669. Is contraindicated if there is a previous history of ectopic pregnancy or uterine abnormality.
670. Is unreliable if the cycles are irregular.
671. Is probably the least reliable method of contraception.
672. Reduces the risk of ovarian and endometrial carcinoma.
673. Improves primary dysmenorrhoea.

Theme: Pupillary abnormalities

Options

A. Marcus Gunn pupil
B. Horner's syndrome
C. Third cranial nerve palsy
D. Iritis
E. Iridectomy
F. Opiate toxicity

G. Aphakia
H. Argyll Robertson pupil
I. Holmes-Adie pupil
J. Glaucoma
K. Medullary lesion
L. Brain stem death

Instructions

For each statement, choose the single most appropriate diagnosis from the above list of options. Each option may be used once, more than once or not at all.

674. The right pupil is slightly dilated, with absent direct papillary reflex but normal consensual light reflex. The left pupil is normal.
675. The left pupil is slightly dilated, with diminished direct and consensual papillary reflexes. The right pupil is normal. The knee jerk is absent.
676. The right pupil is small, with partial ptosis and slight enophthalmos. The left pupil is normal.
677. Both pupils are small and irregular. Accommodation reflex is present but light reflex is absent.
678. Bilateral, fixed and pinpoint pupils.
679. The left pupil is dilated and unreactive, with complete ptosis and lateral deviation of the eye.

Theme: Monitoring of medication

Options

A. Thyroid function test
B. Height in children
C. Serum creatinine phosphokinase
D. INR
E. PTTK
F. Serum amylase

G. Liver function test
H. Auditory function
I. ECG
J. OGD (oesophago-gastro-duodenoscopy)
K. Arterial blood gas
L. Serum ferritin

Instructions

For each medication, choose the single most appropriate investigation from the above list of options. Each option may be used once, more than once or not at all.

680. Simvastatin
681. Didanosine
682. Fluconazole
683. Amiodarone
684. Teicoplanin
685. Warfarin
686. Budesonide
687. Heparin

Theme: Hoarseness of voice

Options

A. Acute bacterial laryngitis
B. Acute viral laryngitis
C. Chronic laryngitis
D. Laryngeal candidiasis
E. Tuberculous laryngitis
F. Myxoedema

G. Laryngeal papilloma
H. Laryngeal carcinoma
I. Sjögren syndrome
J. Ortner's syndrome
K. Singer's nodules
L. Bronchial carcinoma

Instructions

For each case, choose the single most appropriate diagnosis from the above list of options. Each option may be used once, more than once or not at all.

688. A 69-year-old heavy smoker presents with a seven-week history of hoarseness of voice and weight loss. On laryngoscopy, the left vocal cord is near the midline and doesn't move. The larynx otherwise looks normal.

689. A 72-year-old heavy smoker with a long history of COPD presents with a three-week history of hoarseness of voice. He'd been on three different inhalers for at least two years. O/E: the throat is red with a few white patches. Laryngoscopy shows reddish larynx and vocal cords which move normally.

690. A 40-year-old auctioneer presents with a six-week history of hoarseness of voice. He neither smokes nor drinks any alcohol. Laryngoscopy shows slightly reddish vocal cords with a small swelling at the junction of the anterior third and the posterior two-thirds of *each* vocal cord.

691. A 64-year-old heavy smoker and alcoholic presents with a five-week history of hoarseness of voice. Laryngoscopy shows a greyish white swelling at the anterior third of the left vocal cord.

692. A fit and healthy 10-year-old boy presents with a two-week history of hoarseness of voice. Laryngoscopy shows a pedunculated swelling on the left vocal cord.

693. A 42-year-old woman with a long history of mitral stenosis presents with progressive hoarseness of voice over the last few months. Chest x-ray shows a remarkably enlarged left atrium. Laryngoscopy shows normal larynx but the left vocal cord is near the midline and doesn't move.

Theme: Milestones in children

Options

A. 0–2 months
B. 2–5 months
C. 4–7 months
D. 7–10 months
E. 11–14 months
F. 14–18 months

G. 18–24 months
H. 3 years
I. 4 years
J. 5 years
K. 6–8 years
L. 8–10 years

Instructions

For each milestone, choose the single most appropriate age from the above list of options. Each option may be used once, more than once or not at all.

694. Retains head in an upright position
695. Crawls
696. Talks in simple phrases
697. Develops concepts of size, shape, colour, place and time
698. Smiles spontaneously
699. Drinks from a cup
700. Walks alone
701. Rolls from back to front or to side
702. Sits alone
703. Uses words like "I" and "mine", and names common objects

Theme: Prescribing medication in pregnancy

Options

A. Should be avoided as it may affect foetal blood pressure control and renal function
B. Is not teratogenic
C. May cause neonatal Grey syndrome
D. Should be avoided as it may cause virilisation of a female foetus
E. May cause neonatal jaundice and methaemoglobinaemia
F. Should be avoided as it may cause cardiac abnormalities
G. May cause closure of foetal ductus arteriosus and persistent pulmonary hypertension in the newborn
H. May cause abruptio placentae
I. Is a recognised cause of ectopic pregnancy
J. The dose must be halved in the second trimester of pregnancy
K. May only be used in the first trimester of pregnancy
L. Should be avoided as it increases uterine tone

Instructions

For each medication, choose the single most appropriate statement from the above list of options. Each option may be used once, more than once or not at all.

704. Ramipril
705. Danazol
706. Lithium
707. Misoprostol
708. Aspirin
709. Cefalexin
710. Dapsone
711. Chloramphenicol

Theme: Visual problems

Options

A. Bitemporal hemianopia
B. Third cranial nerve palsy
C. Fourth cranial nerve palsy
D. Sixth cranial nerve palsy
E. Cortical blindness
F. Cataract
G. Background diabetic retinopathy

H. Proliferative diabetic retinopathy
I. Glaucoma
J. Amaurosis fugax
K. Optic atrophy
L. Retrobulbar neuritis

Instructions

For each case, choose the single most appropriate diagnosis from the above list of options. Each option may be used once, more than once or not at all.

712. A 70-year-old heavy smoker with a long history of poorly controlled hypertension presents with a two-hour history of sudden onset blindness. Both eyes look normal. Funduscopy is also normal.
713. A 44-year-old man presents to his GP with recurrent headaches and sweating. He noted that his shoes, gloves and ring no longer fit him. He also noted that he tends to bump into people while walking.
714. A 67-year-old woman presents to A&E with a two-hour history of blindness in the right eye which felt like a curtain descending over her vision. Within half an hour, her vision returns to normal. General examination, funduscopy, chest x-ray and routine blood tests are all normal.
715. A 34-year-old nurse presents with a three-month history of intermittent numbness and tingling in her left arm and blurring of vision. Visual field studies confirm loss of central vision in the left eye. Funduscopy is normal.
716. A 56-year-old alcoholic with no fixed abode presents with a three-month history of reduced visual acuity. Funduscopy shows pale discs but the retina seems normal.

Theme: Muscle weakness

Options

A. Hypocalcaemia
B. Hypokalaemia
C. Spinal cord compression
D. Anterior cerebral artery infarct
E. Middle cerebral artery infarct
F. Multiple sclerosis
G. Guillain-Barré syndrome
H. Myasthaenia gravis
I. Motor neurone disease
J. Poliomyelitis
K. Cerebellar syndrome
L. Alcoholic myopathy

Instructions

For each case, choose the single most appropriate diagnosis from the above list of options. Each option may be used once, more than once or not at all.

717. A 27-year-old woman with a history of vitiligo and autoimmune thyroid disease presents with a two-week history of worsening fatiguability and diplopia. Tensilon test is positive.
718. A 79-year-old hypertensive woman presents with sudden weakness of the right side of her body, expressive dysphasia and right-sided sensory inattention.
719. A 64-year-old man with metastatic prostatic carcinoma presents with a one-week history of worsening lower limb weakness, constipation and recurrent falls. O/E: bilateral weakness of both lower limbs (grade 4/5), hyperreflexia, extensor plantars and a sensory level at T9.
720. A 39-year-old woman presents with a one-week history of lower limb weakness following acute gastroenteritis. O/E: bilateral distal weakness of both lower limbs (grade 4/5), diminished reflexes and absent plantars. Superficial sensation is also reduced. The rest of neurological examination is unremarkable.
721. A 56-year-old man presents with a four-month history of pain and weakness of all limbs. O/E: clubbing, spider naevi, Dupuytren's contracture and proximal myopathy.
722. A 62-year-old woman presents with progressive assymetrical weakness of all limbs, dysphagia and nasal regurgitation. O/E: wasting and fasciculation of all limbs, tongue is flaccid and fasciculating and the jaw jerk is absent. There is no sensory loss. Ocular movement and cerebellar function are intact.

Theme: Physical signs in ophthalmology

Options

A. Tunnel vision
B. Bitemporal hemianopia
C. Cherry red spot
D. Argyll Robertson pupil
E. Holmes-Adie pupil
F. Angioid streaks
G. Flame-shaped haemorrhages

H. Homonymous hemianopia
I. Hard exudates
J. Cotton wool patches
K. Heterochromia of the iris
L. Exophthalmos

Instructions

For each diagnosis, choose the single most appropriate physical sign from the above list of options. Each option may be used once, more than once or not at all.

723. Retinitis pigmentosa
724. Neurosyphilis
725. Central retinal artery occlusion
726. Pituitary tumour (macroadenoma)
727. Cerebrovascular accident
728. Marfan's syndrome
729. Pseudoxanthoma elasticum
730. Graves' disease

Theme: Dysphagia

Options

A. Oesophageal candidiasis
B. Pharyngeal pouch
C. Scleroderma
D. Chagas' disease
E. Pharyngeal web
F. Myasthenia gravis
G. Bulbar palsy

H. Pseudobulbar palsy
I. Gastrooesophageal reflux disease (GORD)
J. Herpetic oesophagitis
K. Cardiac achalasia
L. Oesophageal carcinoma

Instructions

For each case, choose the single most appropriate diagnosis from the above list of options. Each option may be used once, more than once or not at all.

731. A 50-year-old man presents with a four-month history of progressive dysphagia, nasal regurgitation and dysarthria. O/E: the tongue is flaccid and fasciculating, palatal movement and jaw jerk are both absent. Ocular movement is normal.
732. A 62-year-old man presents with a four-month history of progressive dysphagia mainly to solids, and weight loss of 8 kg. Investigations show iron deficiency anaemia and hypoalbuminaemia.
733. A 42-year-old obese woman presents with a ten-month history of burning epigastric pain which is worse at night or after oily food. Over the last two weeks she developed occasional dysphagia to solids. Endoscopy shows hiatus hernia, inflammation and stricture at the lower third of the oesophagus.
734. A 35-year-old woman presents with a two-month history of chest pain, dysphagia and regurgitation of solids and fluids. Barium swallow shows beak-like tapering of the lower third of the oesophagus.
735. A 31-year-old HIV positive man presents with a one-week history of dysphagia and odynophagia, mainly to solids. Barium swallow shows multiple oesophageal ulcers.

Theme: Psychiatric illness

Options

A. Post-traumatic stress disorder
B. Bereavement reaction
C. Generalised anxiety disorder
D. Agoraphobia
E. Dementia
F. Paranoid schizophrenia
G. Panic disorder
H. Bipolar disorder
I. Depression
J. Mania
K. Chronic fatigue syndrome
L. Delirium

Instructions

For each case, choose the single most appropriate diagnosis from the above list of options. Each option may be used once, more than once or not at all.

736. A 27-year-old man presents with palpitations, shortness of breath and low mood. He feels "uncomfortable", particularly when he goes shopping. He recently lost his job as a musician and he was finding it increasingly difficult to perform in the presence of an audience.
737. A 53-year-old woman who lost her husband in an accident five months ago presents with poor memory and concentration. She is also complaining of insomnia and unexplained anger.
738. A 26-year-old man reports hearing voices swearing at him. He claims to be closely followed by the CIA through satellites. One year ago he lost his job as computer programmer due to his poor concentration and bizarre behaviour.
739. A 42-year-old woman presents with tiredness on minimal effort with rest bringing little relief. She complains of lack of energy, headache, poor memory and muscle ache. Physical examination and investigations were normal.
740. A 70-year-old inpatient at a surgical ward becomes increasingly confused over 12 hours. He is agitated, completely disorientated and very sweaty.

Theme: ECG findings in arrhythmias and conduction defects

Options

A. Normal P waves and PR interval. Wide QRS complexes with deep S waves in lead V_6.

B. Abnormal P waves. Normal QRS complexes. Ventricular rate is regular at 180 bpm.

C. Absent P waves. Normal QRS complexes. Ventricular rate is irregular at 135 bpm.

D. Saw-tooth baseline. Normal QRS complexes. Ventricular rate is regular at 150 bpm.

E. Normal P waves. Normal QRS complexes. Ventricular rate is regular at 140 bpm.

F. Absent P waves. Predominantly negative QRS complexes in leads V_4 to V_6.

G. Short PR interval. Delta waves. Ventricular rate is regular at 90 bpm.

H. A bizarre and broadened QRS complex followed by a T wave pointing in the opposite direction to the QRS component. The QRS is not preceded by a P wave.

I. Normal and regular P waves and QRS complexes. Constantly prolonged PR interval. Ventricular rate is 70 bpm.

J. Normal and regular P waves and QRS complexes. Progressive lengthening of PR interval followed by one non-conducted beat. Ventricular rate is 74 bpm.

K. P wave rate is 86 per minute. QRS wave rate is 35 per minute. No relationship between P waves and QRS complexes.

L. Normal P waves and PR interval. Wide QRS complexes with inverted T waves in the lateral leads.

Instructions

For each arrhythmia, choose the single most appropriate ECG description from the above list of options. Each option may be used once, more than once or not at all.

741. Ventricular tachycardia
742. Atrial flutter
743. Atrial tachycardia
744. Atrial fibrillation
745. Sinus tachycardia
746. Ventricular extrasystole
747. Wolff-Parkinson-White syndrome
748. First degree heart block

Theme: Interpretation of blood results

Options

A. Old age
B. Anaemia of chronic disease
C. Iron deficiency anaemia
D. Myelodysplasia
E. Folate deficiency anaemia
F. Chronic myeloid leukaemia
G. Alcoholic liver disease

H. Chronic lymphocytic
   leukaemia
I. β-Thalassaemia minor
J. β-Thalassaemia major
K. Cytotoxic drugs
L. Vitamin B12 deficiency

Instructions

For each case, choose the single most appropriate interpretation from the above list of options. Each option may be used once, more than once or not at all.

749. A 59-year-old man: Hb 13.1 g/dl, MCV 105 fl, WCC 6.1×10^9/L and platelets 118×10^9/L. Blood film shows target cells and hypersegmented neutrophils.

750. A 23-year-old woman undergoes routine investigations for a medical insurance: Hb 9.9 g/dl, MCV 73 fl, MCH 27 g/dl, RBC count 6.5×10^{12}/L, WCC 7.2×10^9/L, platelets 290×10^9/L and ferritin 200 µg/L.

751. A 78-year-old woman is investigated for tiredness and lethargy: Hb 9.3 g/dl, MCV 103 fl, WCC 4.4×10^9/L, (lymphocytes 1.7, neutrophils 1.6, monocytes 1.0 and myeloblasts 0.1) and platelets 170×10^9/L.

752. A 47-year-old woman: Hb 9.2 g/dl, MCV 81 fl, WCC 8.0×10^9/L, platelets 440×10^9/L and ferritin 320 µg/L.

753. A 63-year-old man with a long history of epilepsy: Hb 10 g/dl, MCV 111 fl, WCC 3.8×10^9/L (lymphocytes 2.3 and neutrophils 1.2) and platelets 230×10^9/L.

754. A 70-year-old asymptomatic man: Hb 10.6 g/dl, MCV 86 fl, MCH 31 g/dl, WCC 19×10^9/L, platelets 185×10^9/L and direct antiglobulin test is positive.

Theme: Arthritis

Options

A. Osteoarthritis
B. Haemarthrosis
C. Onchronosis
D. Gout
E. Pseudogout
F. Septic arthritis
G. Charcot's joint

H. Tuberculous arthritis
I. Ankylosing spondylitis
J. Rheumatoid arthritis
K. Systemic lupus erythematosus
L. Reiter's syndrome

Instructions

For each case, choose the single most appropriate diagnosis from the above list of options. Each option may be used once, more than once or not at all.

755. A 32-year-old man presents to A&E with a red, hot, tender and swollen left knee. He injured his left knee in a football game two days earlier and 20 ml of blood had been aspirated then in A&E.
756. A 62-year-old obese and hypertensive man, who was recently started on a diuretic, presents with a painful right toe. O/E: red, hot, swollen and tender interphalangeal joint of the right big toe.
757. A 70-year-old man with a 40-year history of diabetes mellitus noted progressive painless swelling of his right ankle over the last few months. O/E: loss of superficial and deep sensation distal to the right knee. X-ray of the right ankle shows gross deformity.
758. A 64-year-old man with a history of haemochromatosis presents with a two-month history of bilateral knee pain. X-ray of knees shows a rim of intraarticular calcification. Serum calcium and urate are normal.
759. A 32-year-old man presents with a two-week history of arthritis, dysuria and dry gritty eyes. He suffered from gastroenteritis four weeks ago.

Theme: Vitamin deficiency

Options

A. Vitamin A deficiency
B. Niacin deficiency
C. Vitamin C deficiency
D. Vitamin D deficiency
E. Vitamin E deficiency
F. Folate deficiency
G. Vitamin B1 (Thiamine) deficiency

H. Vitamin B2 (Riboflavin) deficiency
I. Vitamin B6 (Pyridoxine) deficiency
J. Vitamin B12 (Cobalamin) deficiency
K. Vitamin K deficiency

Instructions

For each description, choose the single most appropriate diagnosis from the above list of options. Each option may be used once, more than once or not at all.

760. Bowing of the legs, lumbar lordosis and pigeon chest.
761. Bruising, epistaxis, haemoptysis, haematuria, haematemesis and melaena.
762. Peripheral neuropathy, loss of short-term memory, ankle oedema, ataxia, nystagmus and confabulation.
763. Gingivitis, bleeding gums, bruises, papular rash and petechial haemorrhages.
764. Sore throat, swollen mucous membranes, oral ulcers, anaemia and dermatitis.
765. Dermatitis, diarrhoea and dementia.
766. Anaemia, memory loss, optic neuritis, impaired peripheral sensation and abnormal gait.

Theme: Bleeding in pregnancy

Options

A. Cervical carcinoma
B. Cervical erosion
C. Velamentous insertion of the cord
D. Ectopic pregnancy
E. Placenta praevia
F. Vesicular mole

G. Choriocarcinoma
H. Abruptio placenta
I. Withdrawal bleeding
J. Bleeding disorder
K. Clotting disorder
L. Endometrial carcinoma

Instructions

For each case, choose the single most appropriate diagnosis from the above list of options. Each option may be used once, more than once or not at all.

767. A 34-year-old para 4+2 presents with painless dark brown bleeding of about 5 cc in volume. She had intercourse one day earlier. B

768. A 24-year-old woman is brought into A&E after collapsing at work. Her last period was eight weeks ago. She's complaining of severe lower abdominal pain. D

769. A 32-year-old Chinese woman, who is 19 weeks pregnant, presents with severe nausea, vomiting and heavy vaginal bleeding. O/E: uterus is large for date. G

770. A 37-year-old para 3+1, who is 34 weeks pregnant, presents with painless fresh vaginal bleeding of about 150 cc in volume. H

771. A 29-year-old primigravida is in labour. Twenty minutes after rupture of membranes, the foetal heart rate drops suddenly. Her vital signs all remain normal. C

Theme: Mode of inheritance

Options

A. Haemophilia A
B. Turner syndrome
C. Familial hypophosphataemic rickets
D. Rett syndrome
E. Marfan's syndrome
F. Leber's optic atrophy

G. Myotonic dystrophy
H. Cystic fibrosis
I. No known genetic diseases
J. Angina pectoris
K. Osteoarthritis
L. Gout

Instructions

For each mode of inheritance, choose the single most appropriate condition from the above list of options. Each option may be used once, more than once or not at all.

772. Autosomal dominant
773. Autosomal recessive
774. X-linked dominant
775. X-linked recessive
776. Y-linked
777. Mitochondrial DNA-related
778. Autosomal dominant with genetic anticipation

Theme: Management of labour

Options

A. CTG monitoring
B. Ultrasound scan
C. Oxygen
D. Oxytocin
E. Intravenous fluids
F. Foetal blood sampling
G. Forceps

H. Emergency caesarean section
I. Elective caesarean section
J. Blood transfusion
K. Diamorphine
L. Regular observation

Instructions

For each case, choose the single most appropriate management step from the above list of options. Each option may be used once, more than once or not at all.

779. A 31-year-old primiparous woman is fully dilated for four hours and has been pushing for 1½ hours. The foetal head is in occipitoposterior position 4 cm below the ischial spine.

780. A 27-year-old primiparous woman is admitted to hospital one hour after rupture of her membranes. She is 39-weeks pregnant but the baby is known to be small for date.

781. A 34-year-old obese multiparous woman presents in early labour. O/E: the presenting part has not engaged to the pelvic outlet.

782. A 32-year-old multiparous woman is fully dilated for one hour and the CTG shows variable decelerations.

783. A 29-year-old primiparous woman is admitted two hours after start of labour at 39 weeks' gestation. O/E: the cervix is 3 cm dilated and meconium is seen. CTG shows evidence of foetal distress.

Theme: Classification of medication in psychotherapy

Options

A. Tricyclic antidepressant
B. Atypical antidepressant
C. Selective serotonin reuptake inhibitor (SSRI)
D. Monoamine oxidase inhibitor (MAOI)
E. RIMA (reversible inhibitor of monoamine oxidase A)

F. Mood stabiliser
G. Typical antipsychotic
H. Atypical antipsychotic
I. Anxiolytic
J. Analgesic
K. Hypnotic

Instructions

For each medication, choose the single most appropriate class from the above list of options. Each option may be used once, more than once or not at all.

784. Fluoxetine
785. Phenelzine
786. Lithium
787. Amitriptyline
788. Diazepam
789. Venlafaxine
790. Chlorpromazine
791. Moclobemide
792. Risperidone

Theme: Neonatal jaundice

Options

A. Galactosaemia
B. G6PD deficiency
C. Crigler-Najjar syndrome
D. Gilbert's syndrome
E. Hepatitis C
F. Congenital toxoplasmosis

G. Biliary atresia
H. Breast milk jaundice
I. Rhesus incompatibility
J. ABO incompatibility
K. Budd-Chiari disease
L. Physiological jaundice

Instructions

For each case, choose the single most appropriate diagnosis from the above list of options. Each option may be used once, more than once or not at all.

793. A full-term newborn becomes jaundiced 14 hours after delivery. His blood results confirm indirect bilirubinaemia and metabolic acidosis. His parents are both Rhesus negative.
794. A full-term newborn develops jaundice at day three, which peaks at day seven, then fully recovers by day 14. His blood results showed indirect bilirubinaemia with normal liver function tests (while he was jaundiced).
795. A full-term newborn develops jaundice at day four, which gradually worsens over the next two weeks. His blood results showed direct bilirubinaemia.
796. A pre-term newborn is jaundiced at birth. O/E: hepatosplenomegaly and congested eyes. Full blood count shows thrombocytopaenia.
797. A healthy full-term newborn becomes jaundiced at day two. His total bilirubin is 10mg/dl. His jaundice gradually disappears over the next few days.

Theme: Physical signs in dermatology

Options

A. Exclamation-mark hair
B. Perifollicular haemorrhage
C. Spider naevi
D. Campbell De Morgan spot
E. Wheal
F. Paper-money skin

G. Nailfold infarcts
H. Yellow nails
I. Calcinosis
J. Onycholysis
K. Erythema multiforme
L. Erythema nodosa

Instructions

For each diagnosis, choose the single most appropriate physical sign from the above list of options. Each option may be used once, more than once or not at all.

798. Urticaria
799. Psoriasis
800. Scurvy
801. Alcoholic liver disease
802. Alopecia areata
803. Cushing's syndrome
804. Ulcerative colitis
805. Normal feature in Caucasians

Theme: Neck swellings

Options

A. Multinodular goitre
B. Sternomastoid tumour
C. Lymphoma
D. Thyroglossal cyst
E. Sebaceous cyst
F. Cystic hygroma

G. Cervical rib
H. Pharyngeal pouch
I. Tonsillitis
J. Bronchial cyst
K. Metastatic carcinoma
L. Teratoma

Instructions

For each case, choose the single most appropriate diagnosis from the above list of options. Each option may be used once, more than once or not at all.

806. A 15-year-old girl presents with a painless swelling in the upper part of the right side of the neck. O/E: 5 cm rounded, smooth, non-tender and fluctuant swelling is felt beneath the upper third of the sternomastoid.

807. A 71-year-old man presents with a painless slowly-growing swelling in the posterior triangle of the neck. He has been complaining of night fever, night sweats and weight loss for about three months. O/E: axillary lymph nodes are palpable.

808. A 68-year-old heavy smoker presents with a painless slowly-growing swelling in the anterior triangle of the neck. He noted that his voice had been hoarse for at least three months. O/E: 2 cm rounded, hard, non-tender swelling deep to the sternomastoid muscle.

809. A 77-year-old man presents with dysphagia, regurgitation of food and chronic cough. O/E: 7 cm soft, smooth, non-tender and compressible swelling behind the sternomastoid and inferior to the thyroid cartilage.

810. A 17-year-old man presents with a painless swelling in the midline of the neck, just in front of the trachea. The swelling moves on swallowing and protrusion of the tongue.

Theme: Prescribing antimicrobials

Options

A. Trimethoprim
B. Cefuroxime
C. Tetracyclin
D. Augmentin and clarithromycin
E. Benzyl penicillin and flucloxacillin
F. Acyclovir
G. Metronidazole
H. Flucloxacillin
I. Fluconazole
J. Isoniazid and rifampicin and ethambutol
K. Clotrimazole
L. Pyrazinamide

Instructions

For each infection, choose the single most appropriate antibiotic(s) from the above list of options. Each option may be used once, more than once or not at all.

811. Pulmonary tuberculosis
812. Cellulitis
813. Pseudomembranous colitis
814. Hospital-acquired pneumonia
815. Urinary tract infection
816. Community-acquired pneumonia
817. Staphylococcal osteomyelitis
818. *Chlamydia trachomatis*

Theme: Chromosomal abnormalities

Options

A. Edward syndrome
B. Turner syndrome
C. Down's syndrome
D. Klinefelter syndrome
E. Patau syndrome

F. Prader-Willi syndrome
G. "Cri-du-chat" syndrome
H. Double Y syndrome
I. Fragile X syndrome
J. Triple X syndrome

Instructions

For each case, choose the single most appropriate diagnosis from the above list of options. Each option may be used once, more than once or not at all.

819. A male neonate with cleft lip and palate, low-set ears and polydactyly. Chromosome analysis confirms a genotype of 47XY (+13).
820. A 17-year-old boy with low IQ, testicular atrophy, gynaecomastia and tall stature. Chromosome analysis confirms a genotype of 47XXY.
821. A male neonate with low-set ears, micrognathia, cleft lip and palate, occipital prominence, polydactyly and rocker-bottom feet. Chromosome analysis confirms a genotype of 47XY (+18).
822. A four-year-old boy with simian creases, epicanthal folds, slanting eyes, short stature and pansystolic murmur loudest over the left-fourth parasternal space.
823. A 16-year-old girl with primary amenorrhoea, webbing of the neck, low hairline, nail hypoplasia and wide-spaced nipples.

Theme: Menorrhagia

Options

A. Physiological
B. Intrauterine contraceptive device
C. Depression
D. Pelvic inflammatory disease
E. Adenomyosis
F. Hypothyroidism
G. Uterine fibroids
H. Cervical carcinoma
I. Chronic alcoholism
J. Endometrial carcinoma
K. Bleeding disorder
L. Clotting disorder

Instructions

For each case, choose the single most appropriate diagnosis from the above list of options. Each option may be used once, more than once or not at all.

824. A 26-year-old woman who was treated twice for chlamydial urethritis over the last two years, presents with menorrhagia and lower abdominal discomfort. An endocervical smear confirmed the presence of *Chlamydia trachomatis*.

825. A 34-year-old woman presents with a two-year history of gradually worsening painless menorrhagia. O/E: she is pale and has an enlarged bulky uterus.

826. A 28-year-old woman presents with a two-month history of menorrhagia. She describes bleeding for five days every 29 days which is of average amount. General and pelvic examination is normal. Full blood count, bleeding time, clotting profile and renal function tests are all normal.

827. A 38-year-old woman presents with a six-month history of severe menorrhagia and lower abdominal pain. O/E: she is pale and has an enlarged tender uterus equivalent to a 14-week pregnancy. She is treated by a hysterectomy.

828. An obese 42-year-old woman presents with a three-month history of menorrhagia and intermenstrual bleeding. General and pelvic examination are unremarkable. Full blood count shows mild anaemia. Clotting profile, liver function tests and ultrasound are normal. Diagnosis is confirmed by D&C.

Theme: Choice of contraception

Options

A. Condom
B. Vasectomy
C. IUCD (IntraUterine Contraceptive Device)
D. Depoprovera (progesterone depot injection)
E. Progesterone-only pill
F. Combined oral contraceptive pill
G. Post-coital high-dose levonorgestrel
H. Laparascopic sterilisation
I. Spermicide
J. Mifepristone
K. Norplant (progesterone implant)

Instructions

For each case, choose the single most appropriate contraception from the above list of options. Each option may be used once, more than once or not at all.

829. A 20-year-old waitress discovers that her partner is hepatitis C positive. She still wishes to continue her relationship with him.
830. A 28-year-old lawyer suffering from irregular, heavy and painful periods attends her GP's surgery asking for contraception.
831. A 37-year-old housewife, who has four children, attends her GP's surgery asking for contraception. She has completed her family. She is not keen on oral contraceptive pills or any surgical intervention and her husband refuses to have a vasectomy or use condoms.
832. A 23-year-old air hostess with a history of migraine attends her GP's surgery asking for contraception for at least one year. Her partner refuses to use condoms.
833. A 20-year-old student had unprotected intercourse two days prior to attending her GP's surgery. She is concerned that she might become pregnant.
834. A 31-year-old smoker with two children attends her GP's surgery asking for contraception. She has a history of left femoral thrombosis and menometrorrhagia. She is not entirely sure if she would like a third child in the future. Her partner refuses to use condoms or have a vasectomy.

Theme: Haematuria

Options

A. Ureteric stone
B. Renal tuberculosis
C. Renal stone
D. Polycystic kidneys
E. Haemophilia
F. Cystitis

G. Renal cell carcinoma
H. Nephroblastoma
I. Prostatic carcinoma
J. Bladder carcinoma
K. Acute pyelonephritis
L. Acute glomerulonephritis

Instructions

For each case, choose the single most appropriate diagnosis from the above list of options. Each option may be used once, more than once or not at all.

835. A 14-year-old boy presents with a two-month history of intermittent haematuria and right loin pain. O/E: temperature is 36.8°C, blood pressure is 180/105 and pulse is 90 bpm. Abdominal examination reveals bilateral ballottable masses in both loins. Marked plethora is also noted. The patient's father was started on haemodialysis at the age of 29.

836. A 54-year-old man presents with a three-month history of recurrent right-sided renal colic. MSU shows aseptic pyuria while urinalysis shows microscopic haematuria. Plain abdominal x-ray is unremarkable. IVU shows an obstructed right pelvicalyceal system and a filling defect in the proximal right ureter.

837. A 72-year-old heavy smoker presents at A&E with painless frank haematuria. He is otherwise fit and well, but reports exposure to aniline dyes 49 years ago. General examination is unremarkable. Renal function and PSA are normal.

838. A 50-year-old man presents with a two-month history of haematuria, left loin pain, night sweating and weight loss of 5 kg. O/E: there is a palpable mass in the left loin and also a left varicocele.

839. A 74-year-old man presents with frank haematuria. He noticed that blood came at the beginning of the stream. He also has a six-month history of urinary frequency, hesitancy and low-back pain.

840. A four-year-old boy presents with a three-week history of haematuria, fever and abdominal swelling. O/E: there is a palpable swelling in the left loin.

Theme: Bacterial infections

Options

A. *Neisseria meningitidis*
B. *Clostridium tetani*
C. *Streptococcus pyogenes*
D. *Staphylococcus aureus*
E. *Klebsiella pneumoniae*
F. *Escherichia coli*

G. *Campylobacter jejuni*
H. *Streptococcus pneumoniae*
I. *Shigella sonnei*
J. *Haemophilus influenzae*
K. *Salmonella typhi*
L. *Clostridium difficile*

Instructions

For each case, choose the single most appropriate organism from the above list of options. Each option may be used once, more than once or not at all.

841. A 63-year-old alcoholic presents with a five-day history of fever, productive cough and shortness of breath. Chest x-ray shows right lower lobe consolidation. Sputum microscopy shows Gram-positive diplococci. Sputum culture shows the organism to be alpha-haemolytic.
842. A 34-year-old accountant presents with a two-day history of vomiting and diarrhoea, following a meal at a restaurant. Stool microscopy shows Gram-negative mobile rods.
843. A 24-year-old A&E nurse presents with severe headache, photophobia, fever and skin rash. Cerebrospinal fluid microscopy shows Gram-negative cocci.
844. A 69-year-old woman presents with dysuria and frequency of micturition for three days. Mid-stream urine microscopy shows Gram-negative bacilli.
845. A 23-year-old woman develops wound infection following an appendicectomy. Wound swab microscopy and culture shows Gram-positive coagulase-positive cocci.
846. A 79-year-old woman who had several courses of antibiotics for recurrent chest infections presents with worsening diarrhoea. Flexible sigmoidoscopy shows white mucosal plaques.

149

Theme: Earache

Options

A. Bell's palsy
B. Ramsay Hunt syndrome
C. Furunculosis
D. Carcinoma of the ear canal
E. Malignant otitis externa
F. Acute otitis externa

G. Acute otitis media
H. Bullous myringitis
I. Carcinoma of the tongue
J. Acute barotraumas
K. Rheumatoid arthritis
L. Cervical spondylosis

Instructions

For each case, choose the single most appropriate diagnosis from the above list of options. Each option may be used once, more than once or not at all.

847. A 74-year-old man who had been a heavy smoker for 50 years presents with a two-month history of increasing left earache, painful tongue and impaired speech.
848. A 78-year-old man presents with a three-week history of progressive right-sided deafness, right LMNL VII palsy and blood-stained discharge from the right ear.
849. A 64-year-old secretary, with a history of osteoporosis, presents with pain and tenderness in the occipital region and around the right ear. She states that the pain is aggravated by neck movement.
850. An eight-year-old boy presents with severe left-sided earache following recent flu. O/E: his temperature is 38.6°C, while his pulse is 120 bpm. Otoscopy shows a bulging and congested eardrum.
851. A 67-year-old man currently under treatment for lymphoma presents with acute onset left-sided earache and left LMNL VII palsy. O/E: extremely tender vesicles in the left ear.

Theme: Differential diagnosis of ectopic pregnancy

Options

A. Ectopic pregnancy
B. Inevitable miscarriage
C. Threatened miscarriage
D. Endometriosis
E. Missed abortion
F. Pelvic inflammatory disease

G. Septic abortion
H. Torsion ovarian cyst
I. Ureteric stone
J. Appendicitis
K. Crohn's disease
L. Irritable bowel syndrome

Instructions

For each case, choose the single most appropriate diagnosis from the above list of options. Each option may be used once, more than once or not at all.

852. A 17-year-old GCSE student presents one week before her exams with amenorrhoea and recurrent colicky abdominal pain. General examination is normal, as are blood tests. Pregnancy test is negative.

853. A 28-year-old woman with an intrauterine contraceptive device, fitted three years ago, presents with a two-month history of recurrent vaginal discharge and bleeding. Over the last two days, she developed lower abdominal pain and fever. Pregnancy test is negative.

854. A 24-year-old woman presents to A&E with severe lower abdominal pain and fresh vaginal bleeding. She admits to amenorrhoea for 10 weeks and a positive pregnancy test three weeks ago. O/E: abdominal tenderness and rigidity, bulky uterus and opened cervical os.

855. A 19-year-old student presents to A&E with severe left iliac fossa pain. Her last period was three weeks ago. An ultrasound shows a 5 cm diameter echogenic structure in the left fornix.

856. A 27-year-old woman, with a history of pelvic inflammatory disease and ectopic pregnancy, presents to A&E with left iliac fossa pain. She reports a little brown watery vaginal discharge.

Theme: Infectious diseases

Options

A. Candidiasis
B. Hydatid cyst
C. Giardiatis
D. Amoebiasis
E. Streptococcal pneumonia
F. Schistosomiasis

G. Toxoplasmosis
H. Cryptosporidiosis
I. Falciparum malaria
J. Strongyloidiasis
K. Pneumocystis pneumonia
L. Ovale malaria

Instructions

For each case, choose the single most appropriate diagnosis from the above list of options. Each option may be used once, more than once or not at all.

857. A 41-year-old man presents with fever and rigors two days after arrival from West Africa. O/E: hepatosplenomegaly. A blood smear shows ring trophozoites.
858. A 39-year-old Egyptian farmer with a history of rectal bleeding presents with haematemesis and weight loss. O/E: hepatosplenomegaly. Colonoscopy shows ulcers and polyps, particularly in the sigmoid colon and rectum.
859. A 29-year-old HIV positive man presents with a three-week history of dysphagia. Endoscopy shows white plaques in the oesophagus.
860. A 28-year-old woman presents with recurrent abdominal cramps and diarrhoea two weeks after returning from South East Asia. Colonoscopy shows multiple colonic ulcers. Biopsy shows PAS-positive trophozoites.
861. A 59-year old man under treatment for leukaemia presents with dyspnoea on mild exertion and dry cough. Chest x-ray shows bilateral reticulonodular shadows. His oxygen saturation drops rapidly on exercise.
862. A 19-year-old student presents with fever and maculopapular rash. O/E: mild hepatosplenomegaly and generalised lymphadenopathy. Sabin-Feldman dye test is positive.

Theme: Regulations for Group 1 drivers

Options

A. Cases are considered on an individual basis.
B. Must not drive for at least one month. May resume driving if satisfactory recovery.
C. May resume driving once cerebral angiogram is normal and satisfactory recovery is achieved.
D. May resume driving only after a head CT scan is normal.
E. The licence must be refused or revoked.
F. Must not drive for one year. A short-period licence may be required thereafter.
G. May be allowed to drive if medical assessment confirms fitness to drive. A short-period licence may be required thereafter.
H. May resume driving only after an ETT is normal.
I. Must stop driving for at least one week. DVLA need not be notified.
J. Must stop driving for at least four weeks. DVLA need not be notified.
K. Driving may continue unless treatment causes unacceptable side-effects. DVLA need not be notified.
L. Must stop driving for three years, then reapply.

Instructions

For each diagnosis, choose the single most appropriate line of action from the above list of options. Each option may be used once, more than once or not at all.

863. Meningioma
864. Angioplasty
865. Night blindness
866. CABG
867. Cerebrovascular disease
868. Hypertension
869. Subarachnoid haemorrhage (no cause identified)
870. Parkinson's disease
871. Migraine
872. Severe uncorrected myopia (visual acuity < 1/60)

Theme: Scrotal swelling

Options

A. Torsion testis
B. Inguinal hernia
C. Mumps orchitis
D. Sebaceous cyst
E. Testicular seminoma
F. Testicular teratoma
G. Epididymal cyst
H. Epididymo-orchitis
I. Tuberculous orchitis
J. Varicocele
K. Haematocele
L. Hydrocele

Instructions

For each case, choose the single most appropriate diagnosis from the above list of options. Each option may be used once, more than once or not at all.

873. A 19-year-old student presents with a 24-hour history of tender left scrotal swelling. He reported that it followed an injury during a game of rugby. O/E: the left hemiscrotum is very tender, fluctuant and does not transilluminate.

874. A healthy 63-year-old man presents with a six-month history of a slowly enlarging scrotum. O/E: the left hemiscrotum is remarkably swollen, tense, non-tender but it transilluminates. The testis could not be felt and the neck of the scrotum is normal.

875. A 10-year-old boy presents at A&E with sudden-onset agonising right scrotal pain and vomiting. O/E: he is apyrexial, the scrotal skin is normal and the right testis is noted to be higher than the left. The patient refuses any further examination of the scrotum because of his pain.

876. A 27-year-old sailor presents with a three-day history of worsening left scrotal pain, dysuria, urinary frequency and sweating. O/E: his temperature is 38.7°C, scrotal skin is red and hot and the left hemiscrotum is tender and swollen.

877. A 30-year-old man presents with a painless scrotal swelling. O/E: the right testis is slightly enlarged, hard in consistency and irregular in shape. Blood tests show remarkably elevated alpha-FP and beta-HCG.

878. A 40-year-old man presents with a painless scrotal swelling. O/E: the right testis is enlarged, hard in consistency and irregular in shape. Blood tests show elevated beta-HCG, while alpha-FP is normal.

Theme: Prescribing medication in renal failure

Options

A. Should be avoided in severe renal failure.

B. Should be avoided in moderate renal impairment because of the risk of metabolic acidosis.

C. The dose should be halved in mild renal impairment.

D. May be prescribed provided fluid intake is doubled, in mild renal impairment.

E. Can only be given with diuretics in severe renal impairment.

F. Should be avoided in moderate renal impairment because of the increased risk of fluid retention.

G. The dose should be reduced in mild renal impairment because of the risk of optic nerve damage.

H. The dose should be reduced in mild renal impairment as toxicity increases with electrolyte imbalance.

I. The dose is the same despite renal impairment.

J. The dose may need to be increased in chronic renal impairment in view of reduced metabolism.

Instructions

For each medication, choose the single most appropriate statement from the above list of options. Each option may be used ONCE ONLY.

879. Aspirin
880. Carbenoxolone
881. Amisulpride
882. Ethambutol
883. Metformin
884. Digoxin

Theme: Investigating vaginal bleeding

Options

A. Full blood count
B. Gonadotrophin levels
C. Kleihauer-Betke test
D. Pregnancy test
E. Thyroid function test
F. Pituitary CT scan

G. Hysteroscopy
H. Ultrasound scan
I. Endometrial sampling
J. Cervical inspection
K. Cervical smear
L. Endocervical swab

Instructions

For each case, choose the single most appropriate investigation from the above list of options. Each option may be used once, more than once or not at all.

885. A 28-year-old woman with a seven-week history of amenorrhoea presents at A&E with fresh vaginal bleeding. An ultrasound shows an empty uterus and normal pelvic organs.

886. A 50-year-old woman on tamoxifen for breast cancer for three years presents with fresh vaginal bleeding. Her last period was four years ago.

887. A 49-year-old woman presents with a four-month history of vaginal discharge and recurrent spotting. She had a normal cervical smear five years ago.

888. A 47-year-old woman presents with a seven-month history of irregular, heavy and prolonged periods. A pelvic ultrasound shows no abnormality.

889. A 25-year-old prostitute presents with a three-month history of breakthrough bleeding. She's been on the combined oral contraceptive pill for three years.

Theme: Prescribing medication in chronic liver disease

Options

A. Should be avoided in severe liver disease or the dose must be reduced.
B. Can precipitate hepatic coma.
C. Should be avoided as it increases the risk of gastrointestinal bleeding.
D. May cause idiosyncratic hepatotoxicity.
E. Is safe in chronic liver disease.
F. The dose should not be changed.
G. The dose should be increased.
H. Increases the risk of hypoglycaemia in chronic liver disease.
I. May precipitate cholestatic jaundice.
J. May be beneficial in the prevention of progression of chronic liver disease.

Instructions

For each medication, choose the single most appropriate statement from the above list of options. Each option may be used ONCE ONLY.

890. Antidepressants
891. Frusemide
892. Sulphonylureas
893. Erythromycin
894. Augmentin
895. Aspirin

Theme: Electrolyte imbalance

Options

A. Conn's syndrome
B. Cushing's syndrome
C. Distal renal tubular acidosis
D. Proximal renal tubular acidosis
E. Pyloric stenosis
F. Addison's disease
G. Hyperosmolar non-ketotic coma (HONK)

H. Diabetic ketoacidosis (DKA)
I. Nephrogenic diabetes insipidus
J. Cranial diabetes insipidus
K. Liver cirrhosis
L. Gastrointestinal bleeding

Instructions

For each case, choose the single most appropriate diagnosis from the above list of options. Each option may be used once, more than once or not at all.

896. A 76-year-old woman is admitted via A&E after she collapsed at home. She has been unwell for four days and her GP diagnosed a viral illness. O/E: she is confused and her pulse is 130 bpm. Investigations: Hb 15.9 g/dl, WCC 12.3×10^9/L, platelets 360×10^9/L, urea 17.2 mmol/L, creatinine 145 µmol/L, Na 151 mmol/L, K 5.6 mmol/L, cl 98 mmol/L, HCO_3 22 mmol/L and glucose 64 mmol/L.

897. A 33-year-old man presents to his GP with a three-month history of headache. O/E: blood pressure is 215/115 and funduscopy shows grade 1 hypertensive retinopathy. Investigations: Na 148 mmol/L, K 3.1 mmol/L, urea 4.1 mmol/L, creatinine 98 µmol/L, HCO_3 32 mmol/L and glucose 4.1 mmol/L. Urine dipstick is negative.

898. A 47-year-old man with a five-year history of hepatitis C presents with shortness of breath and bilateral ankle swelling. O/E: blood pressure is 125/80, JVP is elevated (6 cm), bibasal crackles and mild ascites. Investigations: Na 132 mmol/L, K 3.5 mmol/L, urea 2.9 mmol/L, creatinine 90 µmol/L, HCO_3 32 mmol/L, Cl 96 mmol/L, urinary Na <10 mmol/L and urinary K 60 mmol/L.

899. A 22-year-old man presents with a two-week history of recurrent loin pain. General examination is unremarkable. Investigations: Na 138 mmol/L, K 2.5 mmol/L, urea 3.8 mmol/L, creatinine 92 µmol/L, Cl 114 mmol/L, HCO_3 15 mmol/L and urinary pH 6.5.

900. A 42-year-old woman with a long history of peptic ulcer presents with vomiting for three days. General examination is unremarkable. Investigations: Hb 16.2 g/dl, WCC 6.1×10^9/L, platelets 330×10^9/L,

Na 138 mmol/L, K 2.8 mmol/L, urea 14.3 mmol/L, creatinine 110 µmol/L, HCO$_3$ 36 mmol/L, cl 75 mmol/L and pH 7.52.

901. A 47-year-old woman with a history of pernicious anaemia and insulin-dependant diabetes mellitus presents with weight loss, fatigue, recurrent abdominal pain and darkening of skin. Investigations: Na 134 mmol/L, K 5.8 mmol/L, urea 8.2 mmol/L and creatinine 69 µmol/L.

Theme: Choice of analgesia

Options

A. Paracetamol
B. Morphine
C. Tramadol
D. Diclofenac
E. Nitrous oxide
F. Co-dydramol

G. Diamorphine
H. Carbamazepine
I. Ibuprofen
J. Aspirin
K. Pethidine
L. Colchicine

Instructions

For each case, choose the single most appropriate analgesic from the above list of options. Each option may be used once, more than once or not at all.

902. A 16-year-old man dislocated the terminal phalanx of his right index finger while playing hockey. There is no fracture and analgesia is needed for reduction of the dislocation.

903. A 47-year-old woman complains of jaw pain following a dental extraction.

904. A 63-year-old woman complains of severe shooting pain in her right cheek and around her right eye following an attack of shingles.

905. A 74-year-old man with metastatic prostatic cancer presents with severe low backache. Simple analgesia was not effective.

906. A 70-year-old man presents with acutely painful, red, hot, swollen and tender left knee. He was recently started on diuretics by his GP. He has a history of gastritis.

907. A 40-year-old man presents with vomiting and acute abdominal pain. His amylase is 480 U/dl.

908. A 56-year-old man presents with acute chest pain. His ECG shows evidence of acute anterior myocardial infarction.

Theme: Management of angina

Options

A. Streptokinase
B. Reteplase
C. Aspirin, low-molecular-weight heparin and pain relief
D. Conservative management/observation
E. Chest x-ray
F. Exercise tolerance test (ETT)
G. Echocardiogram
H. Insertion of a pacemaker
I. Thallium scan
J. Urgent angioplasty
K. 24-hour tape
L. CT scan of the chest

Instructions

For each case, choose the single most appropriate step of management from the above list of options. Each option may be used once, more than once or not at all.

909. A 68-year-old man who was thrombolysed with streptokinase for an acute inferolateral myocardial infarction six months earlier presents with a three-hour history of typical chest pain. His ECG shows 3 mm ST elevation in the lateral leads.

910. A 49-year-old heavy smoker presents with a four-hour history of typical chest pain. His ECG shows 3 mm ST elevation in anterior leads. His blood pressure is 110/70 and his pulse is 74 bpm (regular). On further questioning, he has no contraindications to thrombolysis.

911. A 62-year-old diabetic and hypertensive woman presents with a 24-hour history of on/off retrosternal pain. Her ECG shows 1 mm ST depression and T wave inversion in lateral leads. Troponin T is negative, while CK is normal.

912. A 70-year-old man presents with a six-hour history of severe retrosternal pain radiating to the jaw and left arm. His ECG shows 3 mm ST elevation in inferior leads. He has no previous cardiac history and is otherwise fit and well.

913. A 67-year-old man is admitted with acute lateral myocardial infarction and is thrombolysed with streptokinase. Twelve hours later, he remains in severe pain and ST elevation fails to resolve.

914. A 62-year-old wheelchair-bound man presents to his GP with a three-month history of recurrent chest pain. A routine ECG shows 1 mm ST depression and flat T waves in V_5 and V_6. He is started on a beta-blocker and nitrite which slightly improves his symptoms.

Theme: Causes of mouth ulcers

Options

A. Ulcerative colitis
B. Crohn's disease
C. Behçet's disease
D. Reiter's syndrome
E. Varicella zoster
F. Herpes simplex
G. Syphilis

H. Aphthous ulcers
I. Systemic lupus erythematosus
J. Squamous cell carcinoma
K. Lichen planus
L. Stevens-Johnson syndrome

Instructions

For each case, choose the single most appropriate diagnosis from the above list of options. Each option may be used once, more than once or not at all.

915. A 33-year-old woman is admitted via A&E feeling extremely unwell. O/E: she is pyrexial with a temperature of 38.7°C. There are target-like lesions on her arms and legs and severe oral ulceration with crusts. She was recently started on an antibiotic for a chest infection.
916. A 32-year-old Cypriot man with a past medical history of deep venous thrombosis, uveitis and arthritis presents with recurrent oro-genital ulcers.
917. A 59-year-old man currently on treatment for lymphoma presents with severe pain and reduced vision in his right eye. O/E: periocular and corneal vesicles.
918. A 27-year-old sailor presents to his GP with a large painless indurated ulcer in his tongue. It started two weeks earlier as a small papule.
919. A 13-year-old boy, normally fit and well, presents with a six-month history of multiple painful oral ulcers which heal spontaneously within two to eight weeks.
920. A 37-year-old woman with a history of diarrhoea, weight loss, rectal bleeding and perianal fistula presents with two painful buccal ulcers.

Theme: Abdominal discomfort

Options

A. Endometriosis
B. Irritable bowel syndrome
C. Pelvic inflammatory disease
D. Inflammatory bowel disease
E. Endometrial carcinoma
F. Acute appendicitis

G. Ovarian carcinoma
H. Ruptured ovarian cyst
I. Torsion of an ovarian cyst
J. Colonic carcinoma
K. Mesenteric adenitis
L. Diverticulitis

Instructions

For each case, choose the single most appropriate diagnosis from the above list of options. Each option may be used once, more than once or not at all.

921. A 29-year-old smoker presents with a six-month history of recurrent abdominal pain with intermittent diarrhoea and constipation. She denies any rectal bleeding. Her periods are regular. Abdominal ultrasound and colonoscopy are normal. Vaginal and cervical swabs are negative.

922. A 54-year-old woman presents with constipation and weight loss, while feeling an increase in abdominal girth. She admits to bloating after meals. She denies any rectal bleeding. Colonoscopy is normal.

923. A 17-year-old virgin presents at mid-cycle with severe acute lower abdominal pain which resolvs within eight hours. She is apyrexial and all her blood results are normal.

924. A 22-year-old smoker presents with a three-month history of abdominal discomfort and weight loss of 5 kg. She also admits to three episodes of fresh rectal bleeding where the blood was mixed with stools. O/E: raised tender oval lesions over both shins.

925. A 26-year-old woman who was previously treated for chlamydial urethritis presents with lower abdominal pain and fever. O/E: diffuse lower abdominal tenderness, positive cervical excitation test and adnexal tenderness.

926. A 79-year-old woman with a long history of constipation presents with fever, left iliac fossa pain, nausea and loss of appetite. O/E: tenderness and rigidity in the left iliac fossa. Rectal examination was very painful and showed hard stools.

Theme: Medical syndromes

Options

A. Down's syndrome
B. Turner syndrome
C. Klinefelter syndrome
D. Sheehan's syndrome
E. Eaton-Lambert syndrome
F. Antiphospholipid syndrome
G. Neuroleptic malignant syndrome

H. Guillain-Barré syndrome
I. McArdle's disease
J. Goodpasture's syndrome
K. Churg-Strauss syndrome
L. Reiter's syndrome

Instructions

For each case, choose the single most appropriate diagnosis from the above list of options. Each option may be used once, more than once or not at all.

927. A 32-year-old psychotic patient is admitted via A&E with rigidity and fever. His blood results show significantly elevated creatinine phosphokinase and renal impairment.
928. A 43-year-old man with a recent history of gastroenteritis presents with increasing weakness of his legs and right arm associated with numbness and tingling. O/E: absent tendon reflexes. No sensory level is detected.
929. A 16-year-old woman presents to her GP with primary amenorrhoea. O/E: her height is 143 cm, with bilateral ptosis, high arched palate, cubitus vulgus and swelling of both ankles.
930. A 69-year-old man with recently diagnosed oat cell carcinoma of the lung presents with weakness and easy fatiguability. O/E: proximal muscle weakness, particularly in lower limbs, and reduced tendon reflexes.
931. A 30-year-old man is investigated for infertility. O/E: his height is 194 cm, with gynaecomastia and very small testes.
932. A 38-year-old businessman presents with dysuria, sore eyes and buccal ulceration one month after returning from a trip to the Far East. He reports having had a venereal infection after his return.
933. A 32-year-old woman is admitted with deep venous thrombosis for the third time in one year. She has a past history of a transient ischaemic attack, migraine, epilepsy and three miscarriages.

Theme: Seizures

Options

A. Hyponatraemia
B. Hypocalcaemia
C. Hypomagnesaemia
D. Meningitis
E. Cerebral abscess
F. Subdural haematoma
G. Tonic-clonic seizure

H. Complex partial seizure
I. Simple partial seizure
J. Partial seizure with secondary generalisation
K. Atonic seizure
L. Typical absence seizure

Instructions

For each case, choose the single most appropriate diagnosis from the above list of options. Each option may be used once, more than once or not at all.

934. A 17-year-old student is brought to A&E after she had two witnessed fits. History was given by a friend as she was too drowsy. She "went blank" before falling to the floor, then became rigid and started shaking all limbs vigorously. She bit her tongue and was incontinent of urine.

935. A 70-year-old man under palliative treatment for bronchogenic carcinoma is prescribed a diuretic for ankle oedema. Over the next 10 days he becomes more confused, then he develops a tonic-clonic seizure.

936. A seven-year-old girl is reported by her teachers as developing several "funny turns" during which she becomes vague and stops whatever she is doing for a few seconds, then continues again as if nothing has happened.

937. A 14-year-old girl is referred to neurologists after having four fits in three weeks. It always starts by feeling vague (but conscious), which is followed by a phase of anxiety and apprehension. She then collapses, loses her consciousness and starts shaking, which is associated with biting of the tongue and urinary incontinence.

938. A 49-year-old woman develops a tonic-clonic seizure while on a surgical ward one day after a thyroidectomy.

939. A 23-year-old woman, who is 10 weeks pregnant with a three-week history of hyperemesis gravidarum, is brought into A&E after she collapsed and started fitting.

Theme: Red eyes

Options

A. Herpetic corneal ulcer
B. Scleritis
C. Allergic conjunctivitis
D. Bacterial conjunctivitis
E. Viral conjunctivitis
F. Anterior uveitis
G. Pterygium

H. Acute closed-angle glaucoma
I. Subconjunctival haemorrhage
J. Open-angle glaucoma
K. Episcleritis
L. Trachoma

Instructions

For each case, choose the single most appropriate diagnosis from the above list of options. Each option may be used once, more than once or not at all.

940. A six-year-old child recovering from whooping cough presents with sudden-onset painless and red left-eye.
941. A 39-year-old man recently diagnosed with Behçet's disease presents with a three-month history of recurrent photophobia, reduced visual acuity and watery red eyes.
942. A 31-year-old nurse presents with a two-day history of photophobia, reduced visual acuity and severe pain in the right eye. O/E: red and watery right eye. Fluorescin eye drops show a dendritic corneal ulcer.
943. A 62-year-old man presents to A&E with acute severe pain in the left eye with impaired vision and haloes around light. The pain started while he was at the cinema. He vomited twice while waiting in A&E.
944. A 23-year-old soldier woke up with purulent discharge and discomfort in both eyes. His vision is intact. O/E: the conjunctivae are inflamed bilaterally.
945. A nine-year-old child from the Middle East is referred to an ophthalmology clinic with entropion and trichiasis. O/E: corneal scar and upper-lid conjunctiva shows cobblestone appearance.
946. A 60-year-old chemical engineer, who worked in the Middle Eastern oil fields for 18 years, presents with a nine-month history of progressive encroachment of the conjunctiva over the cornea. His vision is still intact.

Theme: Thoracic tumours

Options

A. Neurofibroma
B. Germ cell tumour
C. Pulmonary metastases
D. Hodgkin's lymphoma
E. Squamous cell carcinoma of the bronchus
F. Adenocarcinoma of the bronchus

G. Carcinoid tumour
H. Oat cell carcinoma of the bronchus
I. Leiomyosarcoma of the lung
J. Thymoma
K. Oesophageal carcinoma
L. Pleural mesothelioma

Instructions

For each case, choose the single most appropriate diagnosis from the above list of options. Each option may be used once, more than once or not at all.

947. A 74-year-old heavy smoker presents with a four-month history of weight loss, tiredness, lethargy and recently haemoptysis. Blood tests show hypokalaemia.

948. A 45-year-old woman with a long history of myasthaenia gravis presents with a six-week history of dysphagia mainly to solids. Lateral view chest x-ray shows an anterior mediastinal mass.

949. A 72-year-old retired underground-train driver presents with a four-month history of weight loss and worsening shortness of breath. Chest x-ray shows diffuse pleural thickening at the right lung base.

950. A 48-year-old man presents with a three-month history of weight loss, night fever and sweating. O/E: bilateral palpable axillary and cervical lymphadenopathy. Chest x-ray shows a mediastinal shadow.

951. A 62-year-old Chinese woman, who has never smoked, presents with weight loss and general deterioration of health. Abdominal ultrasound shows liver metastases. Chest x-ray shows a 3 cm shadow in the right lower lobe. Bronchoscopy is normal.

952. A 67-year-old heavy smoker is admitted with acute renal impairment. It is noted that his corrected calcium is 3.19 and serum PTH is also elevated. A chest x-ray shows a 2 cm shadow in the middle zone of the right lung.

Theme: Headache

Options

A. Meningitis
B. Cervical spondylosis
C. Migraine
D. Benign intracranial hypertension
E. Subarachnoid haemorrhage
F. Extradural haemorrhage
G. Meningioma
H. Cluster headache
I. Subdural haematoma
J. Trigeminal neuralgia
K. Giant cell arteritis
L. Tension headache

Instructions

For each case, choose the single most appropriate diagnosis from the above list of options. Each option may be used once, more than once or not at all.

953. A 19-year-old soldier presents with severe headache, fever, photophobia and widespread blotchy skin rash.

954. A 74-year-old man presents with frontal headache, pain on jaw movement and weight loss. He had a similar problem three years earlier which responded to prednisolone. Temporal artery biopsy is normal.

955. A 27-year-old athlete presents with a sudden onset of severe headache associated with nausea and vomiting. O/E: GCS is 8/15 and he has marked neck stiffness.

956. A 41-year-old lawyer presents with a three-month history of recurrent headaches which feel like a tight band around the head.

957. A 49-year-old man presents with a four-week history of recurrent headaches occurring at the same time every day, shortly after going to sleep. It is usually associated with pain around the right eye and lacrimation. There is no aura and each episode lasts less than an hour. The headache is relieved by movement rather than by remaining still.

958. A 24-year-old obese woman, on oral contraceptive pills, presents with a three-month history of morning headaches which are aggravated by coughing, sneezing or straining. She also noted occasional blurring of vision. Funduscopy shows bilateral papilloedema.

959. A 36-year-old woman presents with a two-month history of recurrent severe right-sided headache associated with vomiting and blurring of vision. She feels generally unwell, lethargic and nauseated about 12–24 hours before each episode.

Theme: Vaginal bleeding

Options

A. Endometrial carcinoma
B. Foreign body
C. Ectopic pregnancy
D. Atrophic vaginitis
E. Bleeding disorder
F. Cervical ectropion

G. Endometriosis
H. Cervical carcinoma
I. Cervical polyp
J. Normal menstruation
K. Spontaneous abortion
L. Threatened abortion

Instructions

For each case, choose the single most appropriate diagnosis from the above list of options. Each option may be used once, more than once or not at all.

960. A 62-year-old woman presents with post-coital bleeding, dyspareunia and urinary stress incontinence.
961. A 71-year-old psychiatric patient presents with a three-week history of progressive vaginal bleeding. She is otherwise fit. Speculum examination is diagnostic.
962. 27-year-old woman presents with a very heavy period and passes several blood clots. Her last period was 56 days ago. Her periods are usually light and regular. She is otherwise fit and healthy.
963. A 37-year-old woman with a history of pelvic inflammatory disease and metrorrhagia presents with dark vaginal bleeding and a two-day history of colicky right iliac fossa pain.
964. A 26-year-old woman, who was on oral contraceptive pills for a year, presents with intermenstrual and post-coital bleeding. Speculum examination shows the visible part of the cervix to be red.
965. A 40-year-old woman presents with a four-week history of post-coital bleeding. Speculum examination shows a cervical ulcer. An endocervical smear shows dyskaryosis.
966. A 34-year-old woman presents with a five-month history of menorrhagia. Diagnosis is confirmed by laparoscopy.
967. A 28-year-old woman, on combined oral contraceptive pills, presents with a three-month history of post-coital and intermenstrual bleeding. Speculum examination shows an everted ulcerated cervix. An endocervial smear is normal.

Theme: Investigating a neck swelling

Options

A. Thyroid function test
B. Excision biopsy
C. Digital subtraction angiography
D. Sialogram
E. Ultrasound
F. Direct nasopharyngoscopy

G. Technetium scan
H. Paul-Bunnel test
I. Doppler ultrasound
J. Fine-needle aspiration
K. Full blood count
L. Iodine uptake scan

Instructions

For each case, choose the single most appropriate investigation from the above list of options. Each option may be used once, more than once or not at all.

968. A 60-year-old woman presents with an eight-month history of a slowly growing mass below the left angle of the jaw. O/E: the swelling is painless, mobile and firm. There is no evidence of VII palsy or any neurological deficit.

969. A 77-year-old alcoholic and heavy smoker presents with a six-week history of hoarseness of voice. O/E: there is a hard painless swelling in the anterior triangle of the neck.

970. A 30-year-old fit mechanic presents with a three-week history of intermittent painful swelling below his jaw. The pain and swelling are worse on eating. O/E: there is a little tender swelling in the right submandibular region.

971. A 74-year-old hypertensive man presents with a neck swelling which has increased in size over the last four months. O/E: there is a pulsatile swelling in the anterior triangle of the neck. There is a bruit on auscultation.

972. A 50-year-old woman presents with a three-month history of a neck swelling and hoarse voice. O/E: there is a multinodular goitre but she is clinically euthyroid.

973. A 42-year-old fit woman presents with a four-month history of a neck swelling. O/E: there is a palpable painless solitary thyroid nodule. She is clinically euthyroid.

Theme: Abdominal pain

Options

A. Acute myocardial infarction
B. Gastrooesophageal reflux disease (GORD)
C. Acute pancreatitis
D. Ruptured abdominal aortic aneurysm
E. Colonic carcinoma
F. Acute appendicitis

G. Ascending cholangitis
H. Crohn's disease
I. Sickle cell crisis
J. Acute cholecystitis
K. Mesenteric vascular occlusion
L. Acute ureteric colic

Instructions

For each case, choose the single most appropriate diagnosis from the above list of options. Each option may be used once, more than once or not at all.

974. A 21-year-old woman, normally fit and healthy, presents with a 12-hour history of severe right iliac fossa pain, nausea and vomiting. O/E: guarding rigidity and rebound tenderness in the right iliac fossa.

975. A 47-year-old alcoholic presents with a 24-hour history of severe epigastric pain radiating to the back, nausea and vomiting. O/E: epigastric tenderness and rigidity. Investigations show macrocytic anaemia, leucocytosis, hyperglycaemia and prolonged clotting.

976. A 49-year-old obese woman presents with a 48-hour history of fever, rigors and right upper quadrant pain. O/E: jaundice. Full blood count shows leucocytosis. Abdominal x-ray shows gas in the biliary tree.

977. A 67-year-old heavy smoker presents with a seven-hour history of severe epigastric pain, nausea and palpitations. Abdominal x-ray is normal as well as full blood count, liver function tests and urea and electrolytes. Creatinine phosphokinase is markedly raised.

978. A 76-year-old hypertensive smoker, with a four-month history of backache, presents with acute excruciating epigastric pain radiating to the back. O/E: blood pressure is 85/50 mmHg, pulse is 130 bpm (right femoral pulse is absent, while left femoral pulse is weak), marked abdominal tenderness and rigidity.

Theme: Prescribing antimicrobials

Options

A. Piperacillin
B. Trimethoprim
C. Augmentin and
   clarithromycin
D. Augmentin
E. Acyclovir
F. Fluconazole
G. Amoxycillin and
   clarithromycin and
   omeprazole

H. Metronidazole
I. Clotrimazole
J. Amphotericin B
K. Flucloxacillin
L. Rifampicin

Instructions

For each infection, choose the single most appropriate antimicrobial from the above list of options. Each option may be used once, more than once or not at all.

979. *Helicobacter pylori*
980. Oesophageal candidiasis
981. Pseudomonas wound infection
982. Community-acquired pneumonia
983. Aspergillosis
984. Amoebiasis
985. Vaginal candidiasis
986. Herpetic gingivostomatitis

Theme: Liver diseases

Options

A. Alcoholic liver disease
B. Primary biliary cirrhosis
C. Gallstones
D. Wilson's disease
E. Hepatitis B
F. Portal vein thrombosis
G. Carcinoma of the head of pancreas

H. Gilbert's syndrome
I. Haemochromatosis
J. Metastatic liver disease
K. Autoimmune liver disease
L. Budd-Chiari disease

Instructions

For each case, choose the single most appropriate diagnosis from the above list of options. Each option may be used once, more than once or not at all.

987. A 38-year-old woman, on oral contraceptive pills, presents with progressive jaundice and right-upper quadrant pain. She has a history of deep venous thrombosis. O/E: tender hepatomegaly, ascites, bilateral ankle and sacral oedema. The spleen was not palpable.

988. A 62-year-old man presents with a three-week history of progressive jaundice, dark urine, plate stools and weight loss of 6 kg. O/E: jaundice, but no organomegaly or ascites. Abdominal ultrasound confirms a dilated common bile duct and gall bladder, but no gallstones are seen. The pancreas could not be visualised clearly due to bowel gas.

989. A 36-year-old man presents with a three-day history of fever, productive cough and shortness of breath. O/E: jaundice, but no organomegaly or ascites. Chest auscultation reveals few left basal crackles. Chest x-ray shows left-lower lobe consolidation. Liver function tests are normal apart from unconjugated hyperbilirubinaemia.

990. A 47-year-old woman presents with a five-week history of worsening jaundice and a three-month history of severe itching which did not respond to antihistamines. O/E: 2 cm hepatomegaly, clubbing, xanthomata and jaundice.

991. A 57-year-old man with a history of arthritis, diabetes mellitus and congestive cardiac failure, noted that his skin became darker and he had become more lethargic recently. O/E: 1 cm hepatomegaly, 1 cm splenomegaly and gynaecomastia.

Theme: Carcinogens

Options

A. Nitrosamines
B. Ultraviolet light
C. Human herpes virus type 8
D. Aflatoxin B1
E. Epstein Barr virus
F. Polycyclic aromatic hydrocarbons

G. Human papilloma virus
H. Beta-naphthylamine
I. Betel nut
J. *Helicobacter pylori*
K. Asbestos
L. Ionising radiation

Instructions

For each tumour, choose the single most appropriate carcinogen from the above list of options. Each option may be used once, more than once or not at all.

992. Hepatocellular carcinoma
993. Adenocarcinoma of the stomach
994. Primary lymphoma of the stomach
995. Squamous cell carcinoma of the lung
996. Transitional cell carcinoma of the bladder
997. Papillary carcinoma of the thyroid
998. Malignant melanoma of the skin
999. Squamous cell carcinoma of the cervix
1000. Burkitt's lymphoma

Answers

1.	G	46.	B	91.	J	136.	B	181.	H
2.	J	47.	F	92.	H	137.	J	182.	D
3.	K	48.	J	93.	A	138.	K	183.	A
4.	E	49.	G	94.	F	139.	H	184.	H
5.	F	50.	D	95.	B	140.	D	185.	K
6.	C	51.	H	96.	A	141.	E	186.	C
7.	D	52.	H	97.	C	142.	F	187.	I
8.	I	53.	A	98.	B	143.	I	188.	F
9.	B	54.	F	99.	C	144.	G	189.	H
10.	K	55.	I	100.	A	145.	C	190.	A
11.	E	56.	D	101.	A	146.	F	191.	G
12.	G	57.	J	102.	H	147.	K	192.	J
13.	D	58.	G	103.	I	148.	A	193.	B
14.	G	59.	A	104.	A	149.	E	194.	G
15.	E	60.	E	105.	E	150.	I	195.	A
16.	F	61.	H	106.	B	151.	B	196.	C
17.	C	62.	K	107.	G	152.	A	197.	E
18.	A	63.	C	108.	D	153.	D	198.	I
19.	D	64.	D	109.	J	154.	F	199.	F
20.	A	65.	H	110.	B	155.	E	200.	A
21.	G	66.	E	111.	G	156.	C	201.	I
22.	F	67.	A	112.	F	157.	H	202.	D
23.	I	68.	F	113.	A	158.	E	203.	E
24.	B	69.	K	114.	K	159.	B	204.	H
25.	B	70.	G	115.	D	160.	C	205.	B
26.	F	71.	F	116.	F	161.	F	206.	E
27.	E	72.	A	117.	A	162.	D	207.	B
28.	G	73.	D	118.	I	163.	A	208.	J
29.	C	74.	B	119.	K	164.	E	209.	G
30.	B	75.	K	120.	B	165.	B	210.	C
31.	A	76.	A	121.	G	166.	A	211.	A
32.	C	77.	D	122.	A	167.	H	212.	H
33.	D	78.	B	123.	C	168.	I	213.	C
34.	G	79.	F	124.	F	169.	G	214.	E
35.	D	80.	A	125.	D	170.	J	215.	B
36.	F	81.	G	126.	B	171.	F	216.	G
37.	H	82.	H	127.	G	172.	D	217.	H
38.	A	83.	F	128.	E	173.	H	218.	C
39.	J	84.	A	129.	D	174.	I	219.	A
40.	D	85.	E	130.	C	175.	B	220.	D
41.	J	86.	I	131.	B	176.	C	221.	F
42.	B	87.	D	132.	I	177.	E	222.	K
43.	C	88.	F	133.	F	178.	D	223.	A
44.	H	89.	D	134.	D	179.	A	224.	B
45.	I	90.	C	135.	G	180.	K	225.	F

226.	C	271.	D	316.	A	361.	C	406.	D
227.	D	272.	C	317.	I	362.	J	407.	C
228.	D	273.	A	318.	C	363.	D	408.	G
229.	D	274.	G	319.	G	364.	C	409.	A
230.	B	275.	D	320.	F	365.	K	410.	F
231.	B	276.	I	321.	A	366.	H	411.	H
232.	F	277.	C	322.	K	367.	D	412.	B
233.	A	278.	A	323.	D	368.	D	413.	E
234.	E	279.	C	324.	E	369.	F	414.	J
235.	I	280.	G	325.	F	370.	G	415.	G
236.	C	281.	J	326.	B	371.	C	416.	C
237.	B	282.	B	327.	C	372.	A	417.	B
238.	F	283.	I	328.	D	373.	A	418.	C
239.	J	284.	D	329.	A	374.	B	419.	D
240.	H	285.	B	330.	F	375.	H	420.	F
241.	A	286.	E	331.	A	376.	D	421.	H
242.	I	287.	G	332.	J	377.	D	422.	D
243.	G	288.	K	333.	J	378.	E	423.	E
244.	B	289.	A	334.	E	379.	A	424.	G
245.	D	290.	H	335.	C	380.	F	425.	E
246.	E	291.	H	336.	E	381.	A	426.	E
247.	I	292.	A	337.	B	382.	E	427.	E
248.	J	293.	G	338.	A	383.	I	428.	I
249.	C	294.	J	339.	F	384.	G	429.	B
250.	B	295.	F	340.	D	385.	A	430.	F
251.	A	296.	B	341.	J	386.	C	431.	D
252.	B	297.	K	342.	H	387.	K	432.	K
253.	I	298.	D	343.	F	388.	C	433.	B
254.	G	299.	A	344.	A	389.	J	434.	D
255.	E	300.	G	345.	G	390.	F	435.	G
256.	D	301.	I	346.	I	391.	G	436.	H
257.	B	302.	F	347.	E	392.	A	437.	I
258.	K	303.	D	348.	D	393.	E	438.	B
259.	E	304.	C	349.	J	394.	B	439.	A
260.	H	305.	A	350.	A	395.	D	440.	D
261.	D	306.	F	351.	F	396.	I	441.	G
262.	A	307.	H	352.	H	397.	J	442.	B
263.	F	308.	E	353.	B	398.	H	443.	H
264.	A	309.	G	354.	C	399.	H	444.	F
265.	J	310.	G	355.	B	400.	C	445.	D
266.	G	311.	C	356.	G	401.	A	446.	G
267.	C	312.	D	357.	H	402.	J	447.	B
268.	H	313.	H	358.	D	403.	E	448.	B
269.	E	314.	I	359.	A	404.	F	449.	E
270.	B	315.	E	360.	A	405.	B	450.	H

451.	G	496.	A	541.	G	586.	J	631.	L
452.	F	497.	I	542.	L	587.	D	632.	A
453.	B	498.	G	543.	A	588.	G	633.	H
454.	C	499.	E	544.	G	589.	H	634.	I
455.	A	500.	J	545.	B	590.	B	635.	C
456.	H	501.	K	546.	E	591.	A	636.	E
457.	A	502.	L	547.	D	592.	F	637.	A
458.	D	503.	I	548.	H	593.	C	638.	D
459.	E	504.	E	549.	A	594.	A	639.	F
460.	G	505.	D	550.	E	595.	E	640.	K
461.	B	506.	F	551.	J	596.	B	641.	C
462.	G	507.	F	552.	E	597.	D	642.	B
463.	D	508.	B	553.	A	598.	H	643.	A
464.	J	509.	E	554.	E	599.	E	644.	K
465.	I	510.	I	555.	D	600.	G	645.	F
466.	A	511.	A	556.	C	601.	F	646.	E
467.	F	512.	C	557.	G	602.	D	647.	C
468.	K	513.	F	558.	B	603.	A	648.	H
469.	D	514.	A	559.	G	604.	B	649.	A
470.	B	515.	G	560.	E	605.	D	650.	J
471.	A	516.	D	561.	C	606.	E	651.	B
472.	F	517.	I	562.	H	607.	A	652.	H
473.	B	518.	B	563.	J	608.	G	653.	J
474.	C	519.	C	564.	G	609.	J	654.	G
475.	A	520.	H	565.	E	610.	E	655.	A
476.	I	521.	E	566.	D	611.	G	656.	C
477.	B	522.	A	567.	H	612.	A	657.	D
478.	E	523.	B	568.	J	613.	C	658.	G
479.	J	524.	I	569.	H	614.	F	659.	I
480.	F	525.	I	570.	C	615.	F	660.	A
481.	I	526.	F	571.	E	616.	J	661.	E
482.	G	527.	D	572.	G	617.	H	662.	A
483.	J	528.	B	573.	D	618.	A	663.	I
484.	I	529.	G	574.	I	619.	I	664.	C
485.	K	530.	J	575.	B	620.	C	665.	J
486.	A	531.	J	576.	D	621.	D	666.	D
487.	C	532.	C	577.	H	622.	B	667.	F
488.	E	533.	F	578.	G	623.	A	668.	A
489.	B	534.	G	579.	F	624.	G	669.	C
490.	H	535.	A	580.	E	625.	F	670.	A
491.	E	536.	H	581.	C	626.	B	671.	E
492.	J	537.	B	582.	D	627.	K	672.	D
493.	D	538.	J	583.	F	628.	L	673.	D
494.	A	539.	D	584.	A	629.	A	674.	A
495.	C	540.	C	585.	H	630.	D	675.	I

676.	B	721.	L	766.	J	811.	J	856.	A
677.	H	722.	I	767.	B	812.	E	857.	I
678.	F	723.	A	768.	D	813.	G	858.	F
679.	C	724.	D	769.	F	814.	B	859.	A
680.	G or C	725.	C	770.	E	815.	A	860.	D
681.	F	726.	B	771.	C	816.	D	861.	K
682.	G	727.	H	772.	E	817.	H	862.	G
683.	A	728.	K	773.	H	818.	C	863.	F
684.	H	729.	F	774.	D	819.	E	864.	I
685.	D	730.	L	775.	A	820.	D	865.	A
686.	B	731.	G	776.	I	821.	A	866.	J
687.	E	732.	L	777.	F	822.	C	867.	B
688.	L	733.	I	778.	G	823.	B	868.	K
689.	D	734.	K	779.	G	824.	D	869.	C
690.	K	735.	A	780.	A	825.	G	870.	G
691.	H	736.	D	781.	B	826.	A	871.	K
692.	G	737.	A	782.	F	827.	E	872.	E
693.	J	738.	F	783.	H	828.	J	873.	K
694.	B	739.	K	784.	C	829.	A	874.	L
695.	D	740.	L	785.	D	830.	F	875.	A
696.	G	741.	F	786.	F	831.	C or D	876.	H
697.	H	742.	D	787.	A	832.	D	877.	F
698.	B	743.	B	788.	I	833.	G	878.	E
699.	E	744.	C	789.	B	834.	E or D	879.	A
700.	E	745.	E	790.	G	835.	D	880.	F
701.	C	746.	H	791.	E	836.	C	881.	C
702.	C	747.	G	792.	H	837.	J	882.	G
703.	G	748.	I	793.	J	838.	G	883.	B
704.	A	749.	G	794.	H	839.	I	884.	H
705.	D	750.	I	795.	G	840.	H	885.	D
706.	F	751.	D	796.	F	841.	H	886.	I
707.	L	752.	B	797.	L	842.	G	887.	K
708.	G	753.	E	798.	E	843.	A	888.	B
709.	B	754.	H	799.	J	844.	F	889.	J
710.	E	755.	F	800.	B	845.	D	890.	A
711.	C	756.	D	801.	C	846.	L	891.	B
712.	E	757.	G	802.	A	847.	I	892.	H
713.	A	758.	E	803.	F	848.	D	893.	D
714.	J	759.	L	804.	L	849.	L	894.	I
715.	L	760.	D	805.	D	850.	G	895.	C
716.	K	761.	K	806.	J	851.	B	896.	G
717.	H	762.	G	807.	C	852.	L	897.	A
718.	E	763.	C	808.	K	853.	F	898.	K
719.	C	764.	H	809.	H	854.	B	899.	C
720.	G	765.	B	810.	D	855.	H	900.	E

901.	F	946.	G	991.	I
902.	E	947.	H	992.	D
903.	A	948.	J	993.	A
904.	H	949.	L	994.	J
905.	B	950.	D	995.	F
906.	L	951.	F	996.	H
907.	K	952.	E	997.	L
908.	G	953.	A	998.	B
909.	B	954.	K	999.	G
910.	B	955.	E	1000.	E
911.	C	956.	L		
912.	A	957.	H		
913.	J	958.	D		
914.	I	959.	C		
915.	L	960.	D		
916.	C	961.	B		
917.	E	962.	K		
918.	G	963.	C		
919.	H	964.	D		
920.	B	965.	H		
921.	B	966.	G		
922.	G	967.	F		
923.	I	968.	B		
924.	D	969.	F		
925.	C	970.	D		
926.	L	971.	C		
927.	G	972.	E		
928.	H	973.	J		
929.	B	974.	F		
930.	E	975.	C		
931.	C	976.	G		
932.	L	977.	A		
933.	F	978.	D		
934.	G	979.	G		
935.	A	980.	F		
936.	L	981.	A		
937.	J	982.	C		
938.	B	983.	J		
939.	C	984.	H		
940.	I	985.	I		
941.	F	986.	E		
942.	A	987.	L		
943.	H	988.	G		
944.	D	989.	H		
945.	L	990.	B		

Appendix: Normal values

Acid phosphatase:	1–5 iv/L
Alanine aminotransferase (ALT):	5–35 iv/L
Aspartate transaminase (AST):	5–35 iv/L
Albumin:	35–50 g/L
Amylase:	0–180 Somogyi units/dL
Bicarbonate:	22–28 mmol/L
Bilirubin:	3–17 mmol/L
Calcium:	2.2–2.6 mmol/L
Chloride:	95–105 mmol/L
Cholesterol:	3.9–5.5 mmol/L
LDL cholesterol:	1.5–4.5 mmol/L
HDL cholesterol:	0.9–1.9 mmol/L
Creatine Kinase:	25–190 IU/L
Creatinine:	70–130 µmol/L
C-reactive protein (CRP):	0–10 mg/dL
Ferritin:	18–200 µg/L
γ glutamyl transpeptidase (γGT):	
(males)	10–50 IU/L
(females)	7–33 IU/L
Glucose (fasting):	3.5–5.5 mmol/L
Glycosylated haemoglobin (Hb_{A1c}):	4.5–6 %
Iron:	14–31µmol/L
Osmolality:	278–305 mosm/Kg
Potassium:	3.5–5.5 mmol/L
Prostate specific antigen (PSA):	0–4 ng/mL
Protein:	60–80 g/L
Sodium:	135–145 mmol/L
Thyroid stimulating hormone (TSH):	0.4–5 µU/L
Thyroxine (T_4):	70–140 nmol/L
Triiodothyromine (T_3):	1.2–3 nmol/L
Total iron binding capacity (TIBC):	55–75 µmol/L
Urea:	2.5–6.7 mmol/L
Urate:	0.15–0.5 mmol/L

Haemoglobin (Hb):
    (males)   13–17 g/dL
    (females)   12–16 g/dL
    (pregnant females)   11–16 g/dL
Haematocrit/Packed cell volume (Hct/PCV):
    (males)   0.4–0.53 L/L
    (females)   0.37–0.47 L/L
Mean cell volume (MCV):   82–98 fl
Mean cell haemoglobin (MCH):   27–33 pg
Mean cell haemoglobin
    concentration (MCHC):   31–35 g/dL
Red blood cells:
    (males) $4.5–6.5 \times 10^{12}/L$
    (females) $4–5.6 \times 10^{12}/L$
White blood cells (WBC): $4–11 \times 10^{9}/L$
    Neutrophils: $2–7.5 \times 10^{9}/L$
                                     35–75%
    Eosinophils: $0–0.4 \times 10^{9}/L$
                                     0–7%
    Basophils: $0.2–0.8 \times 10^{9}/L$
                                     0.1–1%
    Lymphocytes: $1.5–3.5 \times 10^{9}/L$
                                     20–40%
    Monocytes: $0.2–0.8 \times 10^{9}/L$
                                     3–10%
Platelets: $140–400 \times 10^{9}/L$
Reticulocytic count: 0.8–2%
Erythrocyte sedimentation rate (ESR):
    (males)   Age in years – 2
    (females)   Age in years + 8
Prothrombin time (PT):   10–14 secs
Activated partial thromboplastin
    time (APTT):   35–45 secs